# FACE YOGA

## with me

## ALEXANDRA PAPANIKOLAOU

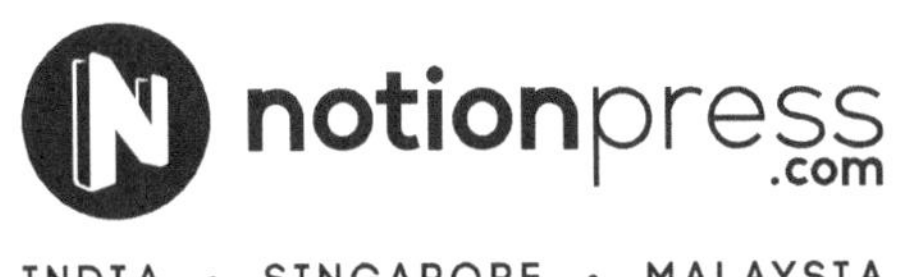

notionpress.com

INDIA · SINGAPORE · MALAYSIA

ISBN 979-8-89026-445-9



Dedicated to everyone who seeks to glow inside out every day

# Contents

## Asanas    113

## FACE MASSAGE    159

# Introduction

## My Face Yoga Journey

It is utopian to talk about your face and how it looks if your soul and mind are not reflected by your body. If your body is suffering from visible or invisible conditions, these are mirrored on your face. Regardless of how old you are, your lifestyle affects your looks one way or another. You don't need an injury or a health problem to look after yourself! All you need is to give this valuable 'You' some free time to feel energetic, rejuvenated, relaxed and strong!

Most people usually start looking at developing their inner self or their physical body after a serious incident or injury, or even a health condition that has transformed their lives or as they grew older. When Covid affected everyone globally in 2020, I took up yoga professionally. I didn't have any serious health conditions. I delivered my second baby in 2021 and was exhausted and swollen. I had the normal pains a pregnancy and a delivery bring. My eyes were puffed, my upper body was in pain from bad posture during nursing, and all I wanted was to do something about it! Although I have been a regular yoga and pilates practitioner for over 15 years, I had studied them to transform my life, body and mind but without a definitive plan. I didn't know that I would eventually write books about my journey and most certainly didn't know that I would be sharing all my knowledge with you, my dear readers. I am doing this instinctively. I let myself experience everything I can with this new path. Here I am today, in your hands, sharing with you some of these experiences, feeling and believing that I can help you and your face look younger.

Paulo Coelho once said, "*The eyes are the mirror of the soul and reflect everything that seems to be hidden; and like a mirror, they also reflect the person looking into them.*" What people usually first see is your face. They will see whatever you feel because this is what you are reflecting. As you grow older, other than valuable wisdom, you will also earn marks on your body and face to prove that you are ageing. Most marks are invisible, but wrinkles, as well as eye ptosis, crow's feet, nasolabial folds, drooping corners of the mouth, double chin, and saggy neck and skin, are visible. Most people can't really do much about them. Wrong! We can work together and with your commitment, you will be able to reduce or reverse some of these signs. Consider ageing as a good sign for your life! Feel blessed for breathing and living a life you can still take control of and work on yourself to transform it into its best version. With face yoga, you can reduce the signs of ageing and look 5 or 10 years younger. This change does not depend solely on how frequently you practice or the selection of exercises you choose to work with. It also depends on your genes, collagen, skin condition, cell production and turnover, hydration, hormones, blood circulation and most importantly your food and water intake. It is wise to add that the daily facial expressions you use and the amount of time you spend in front of your screens can also cause fatigue in your facial, ovular and neck muscles.

# Benefits of Face Yoga

Yoga in general as well as any other form of exercise has both emotional and physical benefits. The extra oxygen intake can benefit your whole body and organs and it will help with more effective blood circulation. As a result, you will feel relaxed and energetic!

## Emotional benefits

**Self-control:** Regular practice gives you the discipline and commitment you need to continue pursuing your goal. The more you practice with enthusiasm, the more you enjoy it and the results will only please you faster.

**Self-confidence:** When you have the self-control to commit to your practice, you will soon have visible results. The results can only make you more confident to achieve this and any other goal in your life.

**Speech improvement:** During face yoga, you work on all your facial muscles. Some of these muscles are used often and others rarely. As soon as you wake the muscles you don't use daily through practice, it leads to clear and more confident speech. Professionals who talk or sing for a living can only benefit from exercising their vocal cords and improving their speech.

## Physical benefits

It facilitates better facial blood circulation which improves the skin texture and leads to a younger-looking face. It reduces the lines and wrinkles in several areas like the forehead, eyes, mouth and nasolabial folds. It also reduces double chin, dark circles, bags under the eye and puffiness, facial puffiness and lifts the eyes and eyelids. It also lifts the corners of the mouth, defines cheeks, lips and face lines, and makes the corners of the mouth along with the eyebrows symmetrical. Apart from this, it improves the skin tone and tones and strengthens the face.

Face yoga is also beneficial for the internal glands such as the hypothalamus, pituitary gland and pineal gland since these get activated through practice and pressure points. The hypothalamus manages some functions such as the heart rate, blood pressure and body temperature, and is equally important to help secrete hormones to manage sleep, mood swings, muscle and bone growth and sexual drive. The hormones secreted by the pituitary gland control our metabolism, reproduction and blood pressure. The pineal gland is associated with the third eye (Ajna Chakra), the stimulation or activation of which is believed to be linked to perception, awareness, concentration, spirituality, mental strength and good vision.

Your skin is the largest organ in the human body which somehow is connected to your digestive system and works as a shield for your internal body parts and organs. It protects the body from harmful pathogens trying to attack it from the outside. Some of these pathogens are viruses, bacteria and fungi, which combined with an imbalanced digestive system can irritate and aggravate your skin with breakouts, sensitivity, redness, black spots, pimples and wrinkles.

Good health is important for a good face. The first step to that goal is water. Water is your best friend for your skin and overall health. Consume at least 2 litres or more of it daily to help your skin maintain its elasticity. Elasticity is important for facial skin since it can soften wrinkles and even remove soft lines. Showers with cold water tone and stimulate your skin. Drinking normal or lukewarm water hydrates and nourishes not only your internal organs but also improves your skin's texture as it increases blood circulation to the skin which in turn makes it look healthier and glowing. Water is a valuable resource for our life and those who have easy access to it should feel blessed and grateful!

Before you start practising face yoga or face massage, some basic rules of hygiene need to be followed. Body cleansing and hygiene are directly and indirectly related to your face and skin. So, when you practise face yoga, either practise early in the morning straight after you wake up after washing your face or just before going to bed when you have washed your face again. It can also be practised at any other time during the day too as long as your skin is cleansed and moisturized.

Always treat your hands with care by keeping both hands and nails clean. Long nails are not practical for face yoga. Naturally, you aim to touch the face with your hands during the day, and any dirt or bacteria can easily be transferred there. While moisturizing or massaging your face use the same product on your hands to soften them to do your face exercises.

Never touch or scratch pimples, especially if you have acne. It leaves scars and no one likes scars, especially on the face. Additionally, there is a big possibility of transferring bacteria or infection to a healthy part of your skin. You have to leave your skin alone, do not put your hands or nails on it. Do not do face massages if you have acne. Follow your dermatologist's treatment and gradually you will see your acne drying out. When you start face yoga and massage, any light marks you have created will heel. You can practise face exercises as long as your acne is not open.

## Cleansing

The washing and cleansing of the face at night are of utmost importance since it removes the dirt stored in the pores during the day. For deeper cleansing, use a cleansing product of your choice. Night cleansing will allow your skin to obtain oxygen efficiently overnight so that skin cells are renewed and repaired to give you glowing and healthier-looking skin.

Morning cleansing is also very important for your facial health. You can choose to splash warm water on your face to open the pores, but always finish by splashing cold not freezing water to close the pores. Overnight, your skin develops natural oils which are good for your skin but also builds up dead skin cells and sebum which should be washed off with clean water splashed on the face.

Splashing your face at least 20-30 times or even 100 times is really revitalizing. It gives you a fresh start for your day, increases the blood flow on your face, removes toxins and brings nutrients to the surface of your skin. Why should you splash so many times? Your skin invigorates to look younger and glowing and this is the most natural way to do so. If you can have your eyes open during the splashing, it cleanses the eyes. This is very good for your eyesight since it increases the blood flow to that area as well.

## Exfoliation

After cleansing, you can choose to exfoliate your face maybe once a week. Dry and dull skin, as well as blocked pores, can be cleansed more efficiently with exfoliation and can give you smoother, brighter and younger-looking skin.

However, if you are experiencing any inflammatory skin conditions it is best to consult your dermatologist for the product and/or method that will work best for your condition.

## Toning

After cleansing your skin, use a toner. If your skin is oily or prone to acne and pimples, your toner will remove any remaining oils or sebum and will work on your skin as an extra layer of cleansing. You can use any alcohol or chemical-free product from your local stores, however, I believe that nature has everything we need to survive, and for that, my favourite toner which is available in almost every household is ice! Ice will tone and firm your skin as well as rejuvenate your skin cells.

If you find the ice too cold to touch, especially in the morning, you can use spoons as a tool. Place some ice cubes in a glass along with a metallic teaspoon and 1 tablespoon. Allow a few minutes for the ice to freeze the spoons and start working with them on your skin, always starting from the neck upwards. Use the same techniques and motions as I describe in the chapter on face massage. The ice will oxygenate your skin cells with immediate effect and will allow better blood circulation to your face resulting in glowing skin. It can work miracles for puffy eyes. Direct ice application several times a day is ideal for open acne as it soothes the popped pimples and reduces swelling and inflammation.

## Moisturizing

After toning, the next step is moisturizing, which will hydrate the skin and support the generation of new cells. The product you use should feel light in texture so it allows your skin to breathe. To apply, start from your chest, move to the front and back of the neck with upward movements so you can lift your skin, then move to the jaw, nose, cheeks, around the eyes and lastly the forehead. After you finish, start tapping your face with your fingers to help your product penetrate your skin. Applying moisturizer daily by using the face massage techniques is useful, but it should be done with a maximum of 3-4 strokes.

## Sunscreen

Even if you are too busy or careless about your skin, you have to use sunscreen daily to protect yourself from the sun and UVA rays which age it. You can apply the sunscreen with the same moves you apply your moisturizer and tap at the end for the product of your choice to penetrate the skin. Like the moisturizer, the sunscreen also should feel light on your skin, so that it works to your benefit allowing your skin cells to breathe. A thicker sunscreen will not work as a better protective layer. It will only block your cells, as it attracts and absorbs dust, atmospheric dirt and pollution to your face.

## How to carry out your skincare routine

In any case, your facial skincare ritual should include at least cleansing, toning and moisturizing. Follow these steps:

1. Blow your cheeks and splash cold water. Blowing the cheeks expands the skin in that area and the pores become clean more efficiently along with the splashing water. Repeat that at least 20-30 times; blow the cheeks, splash, and release. While doing so, keep breathing normally. There is no need to hold your breath.

2. No matter which soap or facewash you use as per your skin type, lather it very nicely over your entire face and then massage it into every corner of your face as well as the neck and behind the ears. Be cautious about the eye area to avoid any eye irritation. Keep massaging for 1 minute to let it work on your skin.

3.  Repeat by splashing cold water to rinse off the soap. Blow your cheeks again and splash water at least 20-30 times or until you feel your skin and pores are clean from the product you used. If you feel splashing is not working efficiently for you at this stage, you may clean with gentle moves and fresh, cold and clean water.

4.  With a towel or tissue paper gently dry the face. Do not use hard moves to dry your skin, just pat it gently.

5.  After 1 to 3 minutes, apply your preferred toner. The toner is a very important step in this process. It needn't be a branded product. It can be rose water or even ice which is commonly available in most households.

6.  After 1 to 3 minutes, apply your moisturizer. While doing this, you can massage the face. I will show you how in the following chapters.

7.  Allow the moisturizer to get absorbed for 2 to 3 minutes, and then apply your sunscreen. It is absolutely necessary to apply sunscreen at least 20-30 minutes before going out in the sun. The sunscreen will protect your skin from the sun but be cautious! Before buying an expensive one, try to get a sample first and test it on your skin. If it feels sticky or any irritation appears, you will know that this is not the right product for your skin type. In most stores and pharmacies nowadays you can consult the beautician and find which one is best for your skin type, just like your moisturizer and make-up.

8.  Apply your make-up if you are using any and you are ready to go. Allow 3 to 5 minutes before doing so, so that your sunscreen is absorbed by your skin.

9.  Repeat steps 1 to 6 once you are back home at the end of your day. Cleansing your face is very important because the sunscreen which is usually thicker in texture works as a protection against dust. The thick product in combination with the dust from the outer environment easily blocks pores and this is where blackheads and spots may start developing on your face.

# Skincare routine

## Day

Gentle
cleanser

Toner

Moisturizer/
Day Cream

Sunscreen

## Night

Cleanser

Toner

Moisturizer/
Night Cream

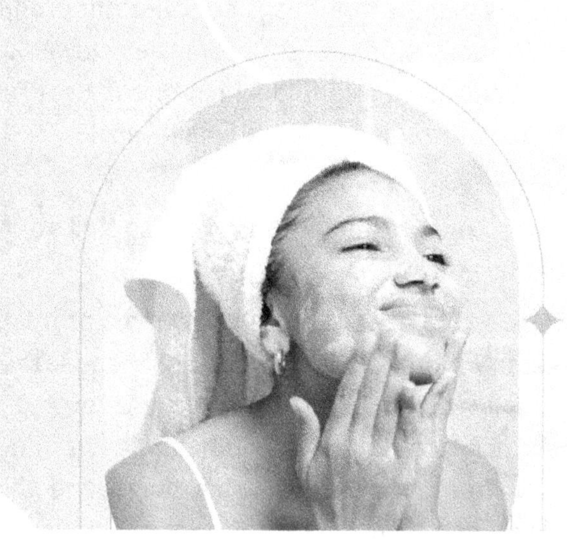

In the following chapters, I will focus on the following:

- Face exercises for all specific areas such as the forehead, the eyes, the cheek and nasolabial folds, the mouth and lips, the neck and jawline.

- Asanas which include ones for warm-up and cool-down, as well as selected asanas from Hatha yoga that will help you not only with your physical body but your face as well.

- Face massage with the help of your fingers and hands that will push the lymphatic drainage back into the bloodstream and relieve you from bags under the eyes, puffiness and facial bloating. The increased blood flow to the skin and muscles will lead to healthier and firmer-looking skin.

Our intuition is always our best companion! I always encourage all my students to listen to their bodies and practice within their limits. When I talk about asanas, it is common for me to say, "Do not do it if it doesn't feel right!"

In the case of face exercises, we aim to stretch and lift the skin, not break it. Our facial skin is sensitive, and the pressure you apply should be tolerable and gentle at the same time. If you feel you need to moisturize your face and lips more during practice, do that so that you further nourish these areas and practise more efficiently.

Regardless, face yoga is a harmless way of exercising and is safe for all. However, if you experience skin-related conditions, consult a dermatologist for a specialized opinion. If you have arthritis or back, shoulder and neck-related conditions, consult a specialist before beginning. If needed, you can practise while seated. You can even choose to support your elbows on a table in front of you.

Your mirror is also a necessary tool for your practice. By looking at it, you will be able to see and correct your poses to achieve a symmetrical result. Also, the only exercise I recommend for unlimited practice daily, even during practising face exercises is this—smile! While you see your reflection in your mirror, remind yourself to keep smiling. Show your teeth or keep your lips closed, but keep smiling! It will help lift the corners of your mouth. But most importantly, it secretes hormones like endorphins, dopamine and serotonin which provide relief from mild pain, fight stress and act as antidepressants.

## Frequency

The two most common questions I face are—how often and for how long? The answer is simple! Whatever you practice, you should do it as often and for as long as it feels good and comfortable. The moment you force yourself, you will lose interest.

However, my principle is to practise daily for at least 20-30 minutes. The face exercises need not be done in a set environment. Your face and lips need to be moisturized and you need to commit to practise the exercises daily. You can start with 5 minutes in the morning, 5 minutes at night when you brush your teeth and wash your face, during your shower, while working or doing your household chores, driving or walking.

Your frequency and duration depend on your motivation for the results you seek. Even 10 minutes of daily practice will give you some visible results in a month. The only thing you need to do is start practising. It is never too early or too late to work on yourself! If you want to add some laughter during your practice, you can practise with a partner.

## Results

When I will see the results? Like with any other exercise, to see permanent results you need to give it time. As you cannot have a six-pack overnight, you cannot reduce your double chin or wrinkles unless you exercise daily with commitment.

The facial muscles are mostly controlled by the facial nerves which differentiate them from the other muscles in our body that are controlled by our bones. This makes it easier to manipulate facial muscles with face yoga. With daily practice, you can obtain visible results in less than a month. However, for a more permanent effect, you will need to practise daily for at least 6 months or longer, depending on your genes, skin condition, age and lifestyle.

To keep a reference of your progress, start by clicking a selfie before your first practice and take another for every month that you continue practising. Look at the evidence of the positive changes on your face as time passes.

As we all know, a balanced diet is the ultimate goal for everyone's life and well-being. Life in the 21st century is stressful and tiring. Sometimes, 24 hours in a day may seem insufficient. Regardless, 6 cardinal principles affect our nutrition which should be prioritised in your lifestyle.

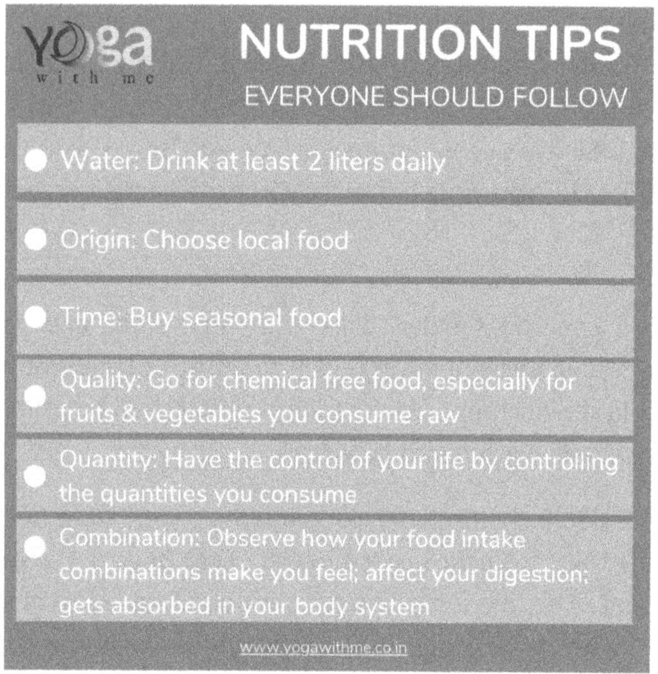


Avoid drinking cold water, as cold drinks or intake of cold food contracts the pores of the intestines which affects the stomach and pancreas and slows them down, reducing the production of digestive enzymes. Enzymes are important to help break down the carbohydrates, proteins and fats from the food we consume.

Feeling your body will lead you to conscious living. Observe what happens to your body when you eat something you are not supposed to or you are not used to eating! Eventually, everything you suffer from shows on your face! Change your habits to change your life!

# Face Exercises

Before starting your face exercises, don't forget to wash and moisturize your face and lips. The following exercises are to be practised daily. You just need to choose which of these suits your needs. Practising these exercises will only benefit you on an emotional and physical level. Results in some cases will be visible even after 1 or 2 practice sessions. Obviously, if you stop practising, the results will start fading!

The first 3 exercises can benefit everyone. Even if you do nothing else, at least practise these 3—Smile, Wow!, and Vowels.

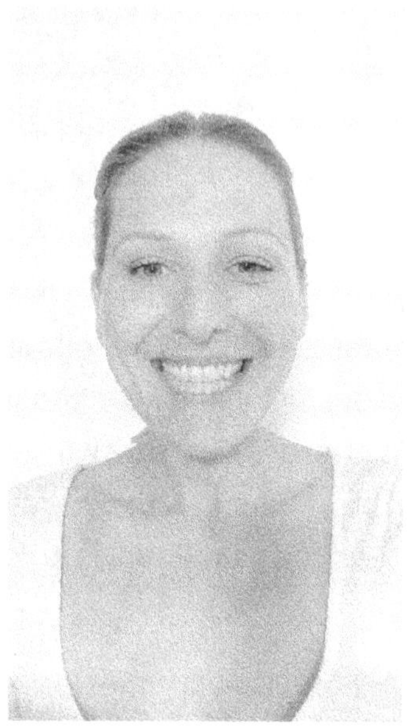

Smile widely with all your teeth out, or with your mouth slightly open or closed. Smile as much as you can during your day. Start by smiling every morning at your mirror! To practise, hold your smile for 10 seconds and release. Repeat 10 times.

**Benefits:** Smiling exercises the cheek muscles and increases blood circulation. Due to this, the face shines. It also creates a pinkish colour on the cheeks, a natural blush which makes you look even more beautiful! It also secretes the hormone serotonin which acts as an antidepressant, the hormone endorphin which acts as a mild pain reliever and increases neuropeptides which relieve your stress. Smile!

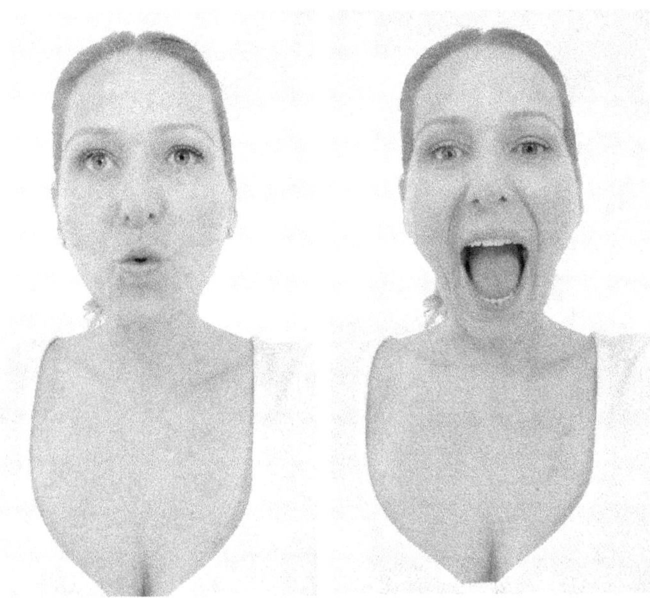

Vocalize 'Wow!' in slow motion in an exaggerated manner as you widely open your mouth. On every vocal, hold the position for 3 seconds. Repeat 10 times.

**Benefits:** This will help you get stress relief and release tension from your facial muscles.

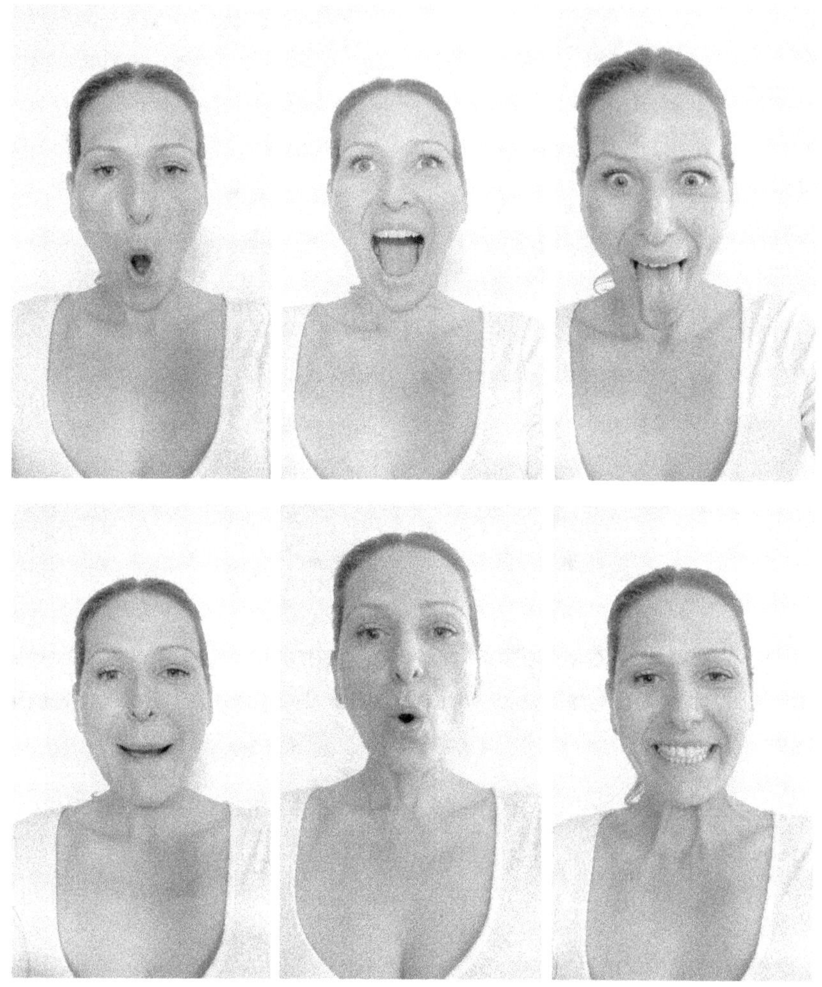

Focus on exercising the sounds of each vowel, by moving the lips to the sound of each vowel in a theatrical way, by overstretching the opening of the 'O', 'A', 'E', 'U', and 'I'. Keep your forehead always relaxed, breathe normally and practice 5-10 times:

- O: Open your mouth, drop your jaw, make an 'O' shape by pressing the upper lip against your teeth and gaze towards the sky. Involving the eyes in this exercise will work on smoothening the nasolabial folds and the puffiness under the eyes. With this exercise, you will increase blood flow to your face and neck. Before vocalizing the 'A', lower your eyes to the neutral position.

- A: Open your mouth wide and make the 'Aaa' sound. You can look up at the sky to tone your eyes as well as your cheeks and neck. For a bigger neck stretch, take your tongue out. Feel the motion in your cheeks, mouth and jawline.

- E: Open your mouth, round your lips over your teeth and lift the corners of your mouth. Make the 'Eee' sound to help you focus on the exercise. With this exercise, you will lift the cheeks and the corners of the mouth as well as reduce the nasolabial folds.

- U: Open your mouth, lift your chin, make the 'U' shape, pull together your lips by bringing the cheeks closer to your teeth, like a smooch, and gaze towards the sky keeping the lips firm. Before vocalizing the 'I', lower your eyes to the neutral position.

- I: With your lips open and teeth visible, stretch your mouth to smile and make the 'Iii' sound to tone your cheeks and lift your lips. Engage your throat to tone the neck and jawline to reduce the double chin.

Close your eyes for a few seconds and smile to relax the facial muscles.

**Benefits:** Increases blood circulation to the face and neck and tones the bags under the eyes. It also lengthens a rounded face, smoothens the nasolabial folds, and lifts and strengthens the cheeks and the corners of the mouth. It improves the definition of the cheeks and makes them seem fuller and shapes lips to give them a brighter colour. Practise by recreating the sound of each vowel without rushing. Stay on each vowel for at least 5 seconds. When engaging your throat during any practice, the neck muscles are toned. This helps in reducing the double chin and shaping the jawline.

**Note:** Make sure your forehead is relaxed during practice.

With the following exercises and pressure points, you will be able to relax and tone your forehead muscles. This will soften and reduce wrinkles or expression lines in this area. Since the position of the arms for these exercises is to be bent at the elbows with the chest open, these exercises tone the torso too.

It is important to avoid any wrinkling on your forehead during your day as well as during your practice sessions. Keep your shoulders relaxed. If at any point during these exercises your skin feels overstretched, stop, apply some more moisturizer and continue.

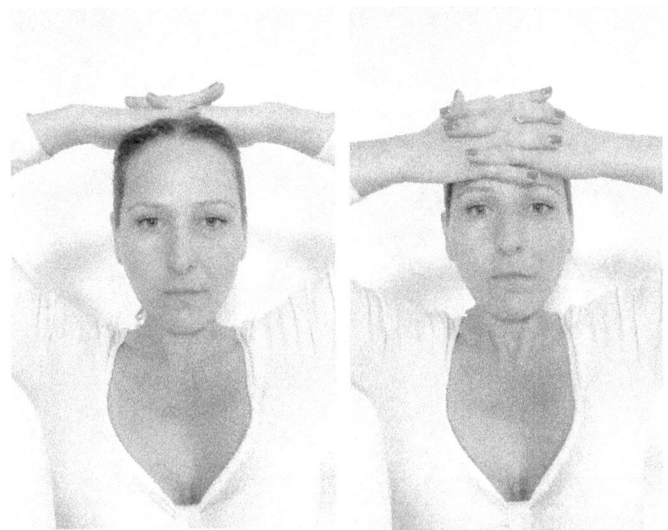

Interlock your fingers and place them on your crown. Start by applying firm pressure on the crown for 1 to 2 seconds and then release. Repeat 5-10 times. Then, with the fingers interlocked on the crown, apply firm pressure and move your hands backwards and forward, like a vibration, 10 times. Continue the same from side to side 10 times.

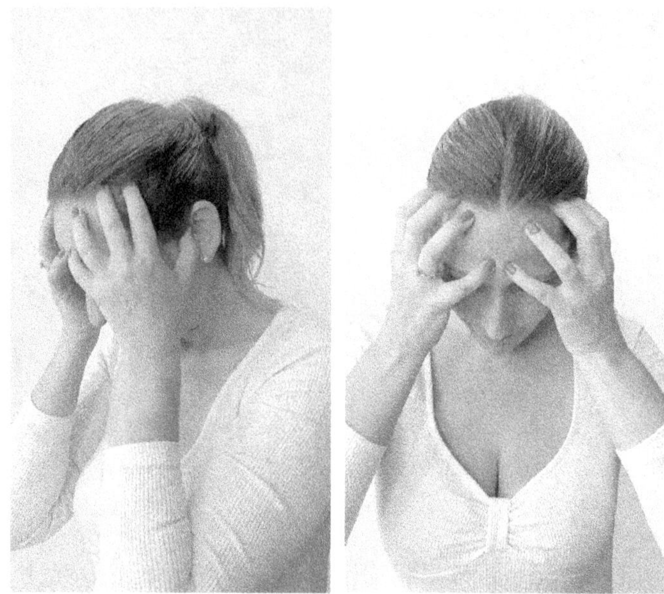

Relax your neck, shoulders and forehead. Place all 10 fingertips along your forehead and apply some pressure to lift your skin. Tilt your face down in an attempt to be parallel to the ground. That way, you will help blood circulation to the forehead and the whole face. Hold the position for 10 seconds while breathing normally. Return your head to the neutral position. Repeat 5-10 times.

**Benefits:** Relaxes and lifts your forehead. It also stimulates blood circulation to your face for a better skin tone and texture.

**Note:** If you experience any dizziness at the end of the exercise, practise the palming exercise or drink some water. Take a few breaths and continue.

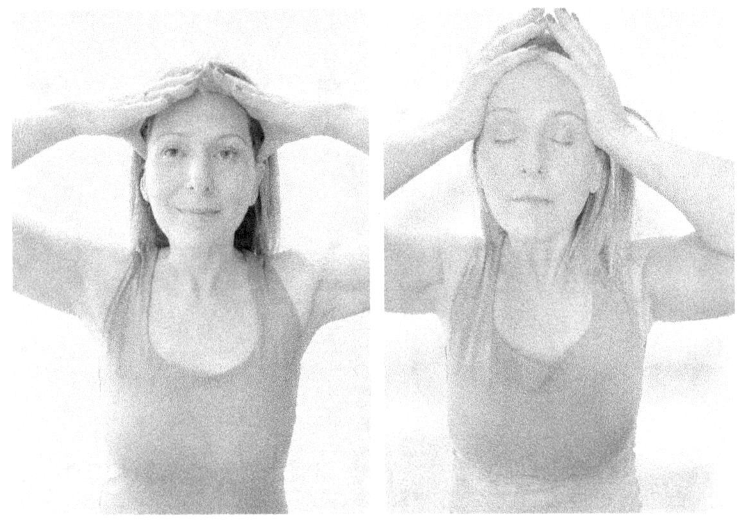

Place your palms like a pyramid with your thumbs beside the top of your ears. Maintain the pyramid by placing your index fingers above the eyebrows. With firm pressure stroke up toward your hairline by engaging the rest of the fingers as you move up. When you reach the hairline, your pinky finger should reach to lift the skin. Slightly lift your hands from your head and bring them back to the eyebrows to repeat the stroke in an upward direction again. Make sure your forehead is relaxed, your chest and elbows are open, and your head is in a neutral position. On the last stroke, hold the position on the hairline for 10 seconds and feel the lift. Repeat 5-10 times.

**Benefits:** Relaxes and lifts your forehead.

**Note:** If the pyramid stroke is confusing while keeping your fingers engaged, you can interlock your fingers on the forehead like in a forehead massage. When you reach the hairline, the pinky finger should hold the skin up. On every repetition, alternate the top hand as you interlock your fingers to support skin lifting on both sides.

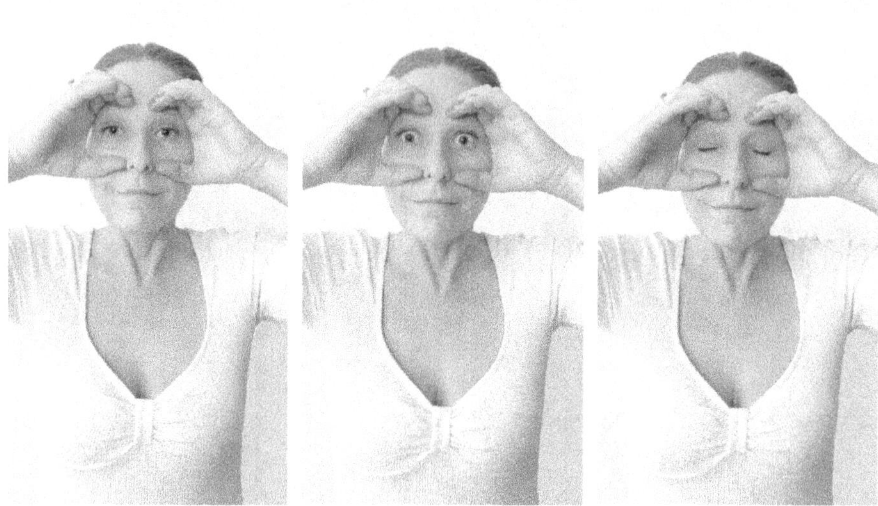

Make a C-shape with your hands above your eyebrows and beside the nostrils. With your index fingers pull your forehead muscles upward. Adjust your position to relax your shoulder blades and open your chest to make it easier for the flow of oxygen. Widen your eyes for a few seconds and then close them. Keep your forehead and eyebrows still. Repeat 5-10 times.

**Benefits:** Prevents expression or ageing lines on your forehead and stimulates the eye muscles. Lifts the eyelids and eyebrows.

These exercises can be beneficial to those who wear spectacles or contact lenses as they will help the ocular muscles function better. Do practise these exercises if you have myopia, presbyopia or a squint. Those with diseases such as glaucoma, trachoma, cataract, retinal detachment, retinal artery or vein thrombosis, iritis, keratitis, and conjunctivitis or those who have had an ocular surgery a minimum of 2 years ago should consult their ophthalmologist before practising the exercises that involve eye movement.

The eye muscles and skin around them are usually exercised by smiling, narrowing the eyes or looking sideways. Such movements make the sensitive skin of the eyes vulnerable to wrinkles. Drooping eyelids, puffiness and dark circles appear with age or with unbalanced life habits. Practise these exercises to sustain a youthful appearance.

These eye exercises should ideally be practised either early in the morning when you wake up and/or in the evening without wearing your spectacles or contact lenses and in a comfortable seated position (in a chair, in a cross-legged position or base position, also known as Prarambik Sthiti). Keep your whole face relaxed during every exercise.

It is recommended before starting to splash cold water on your face and eyes at least 10-15 times to increase blood circulation and tone them up. Moisturize your skin before practice and be delicate and gentle with your hand movements. You only need to lift your eyes and skin, not break it. After practising these exercises, you may feel some discomfort which is normal, since you are waking these muscles up. Splash some cold water and blink to remove the tension or practise palming if needed. Rest with your eyes closed for half a minute.

Half lotus pose (Ardha Padmasana)        Staff pose (Dandasana)

If you practise the eye asanas alone, upon completion, lie in Shavasana for a few minutes if you like.

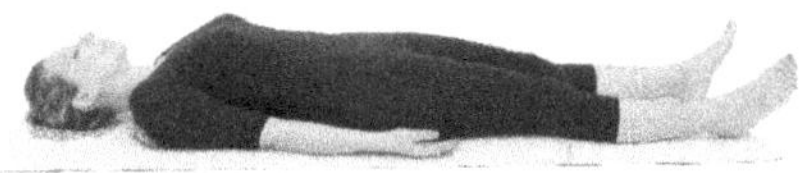

Corpse pose (Shavasana)

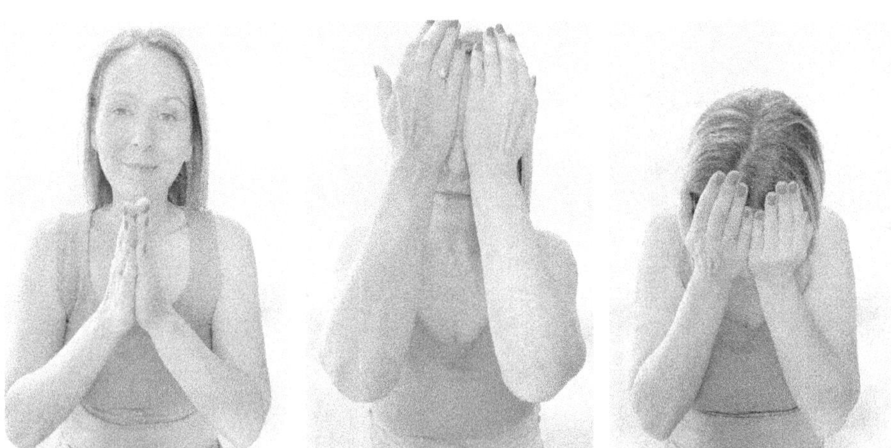

With your eyes closed, rub your palms together vigorously to generate heat and gently cup them over your eyes (the fingers should be above the level of the eyebrows). When the heat from the hands has been transmitted completely to the eyes, lower your hands and slowly open them.

**Alternative:** When performed at the end of relaxation, cup the eyes for a few seconds and while your palms are still warm, transfer that heat to the rest of your face, neck, shoulders, chest, rib cage, back, and wherever you can reach.

**Benefits:** All your energy and heat return to your body through your eyes. Your ocular muscles get relaxed instantly. The energy produced creates a dark space which is important to bring calmness and relaxation. Focus on your breathing and enjoy the stillness of this moment.

**Note:** This exercise can be done in the beginning, in between or at the end of your practice.

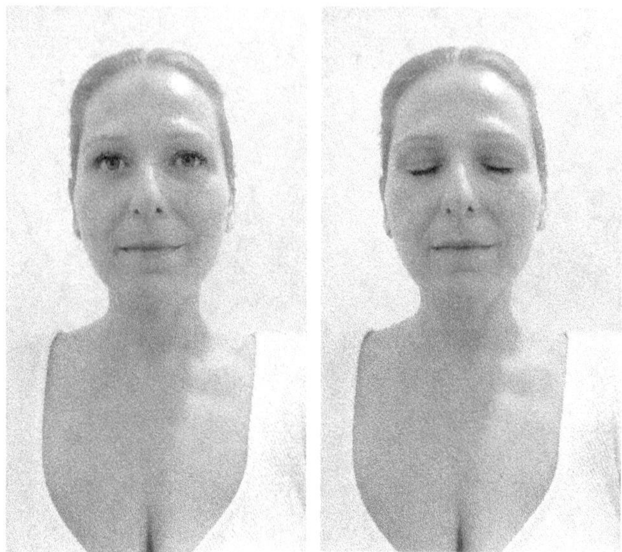

Start with your eyes open and blink them quickly at least 20 times. Close your eyes for 5 seconds. Repeat 5-10 times.

**Benefits:** Those who blink irregularly and unnaturally can relax the eye muscles with this intentional blinking and train them to blink naturally. For the general public, this exercise is a warm-up.

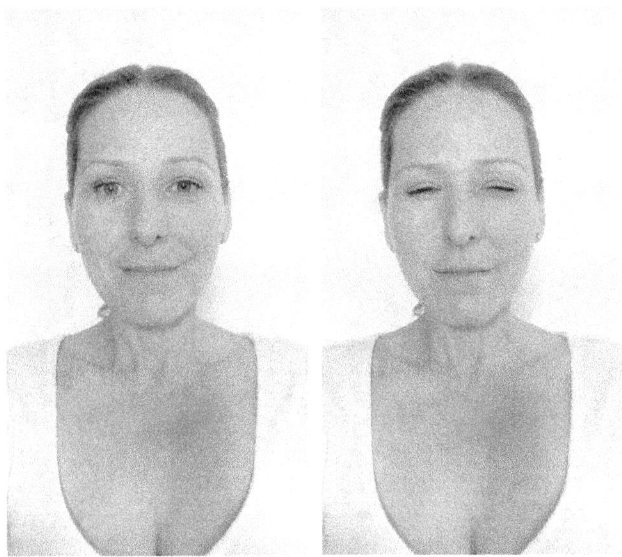

Gaze at a distant point, straight in front of you at eye level and focus there for 5 seconds. Then, tighten your gaze by narrowing your eyes for 5 seconds. Close your eyes for 5 seconds. Repeat 5-10 times.

**Benefits:** Tones and strengthens the ovular muscles and the muscles around the eyes.

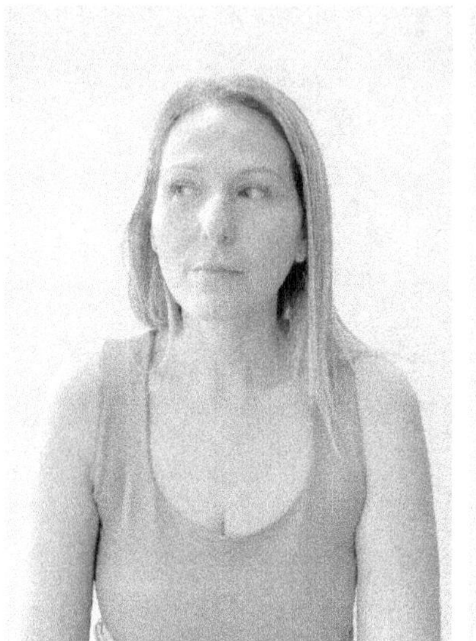 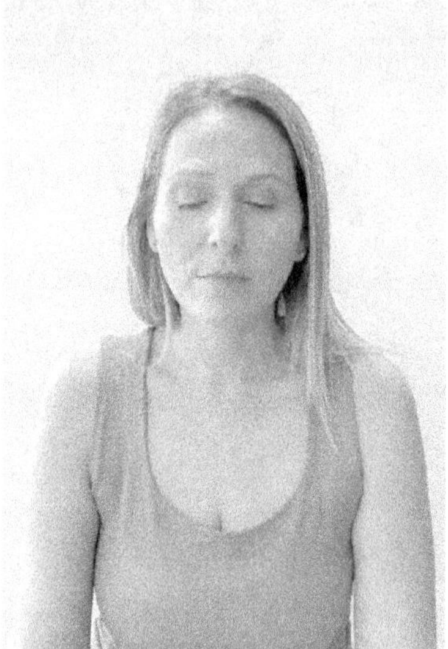

From a seated position, fix your gaze at a point directly in front of your eyes, at eye level. Inhale while keeping your head still in a neutral position. Exhale and gaze to the left. Inhale and gaze at your nose. You can practise one side at a time to avoid vertigo and repeat the same with the right side. This is 1 cycle. Repeat 5-10 times. At any point after completing a cycle, you can palm the eyes if needed.

**Benefits:** If your work or your daily habits involve constant screen time, reading and any type of strenuous work, the muscles in the eye become tense. Viewing sideways relaxes this tension and also prevents and corrects squint. It improves the coordination of the medial and lateral muscles of the eyeball and reduces puffiness and bags under the eyes.

# Exercise 12:   Viewing up and down

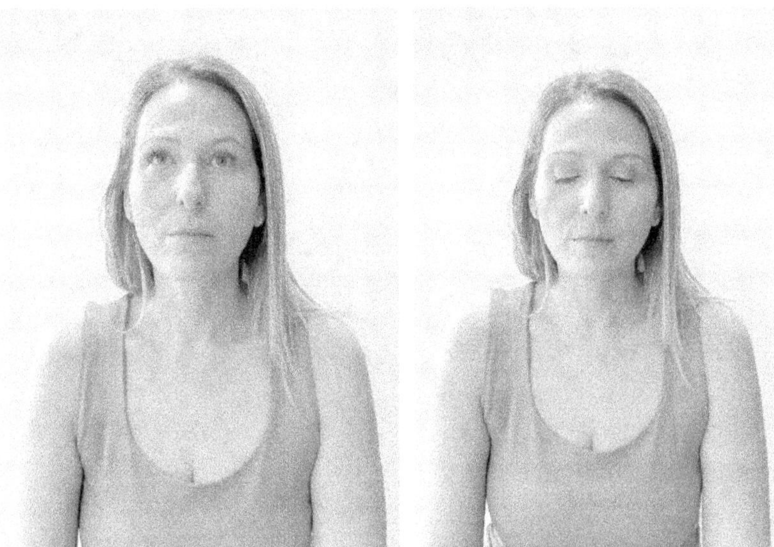

Practise viewing up and down like picturing a clock. Without wrinkling your forehead, start moving your eyes up as you inhale, and upon exhaling, look down (half past). You can practise this exercise either as a continuous and steady eye movement or with a short pause between the moves. Repeat 5-10 times.

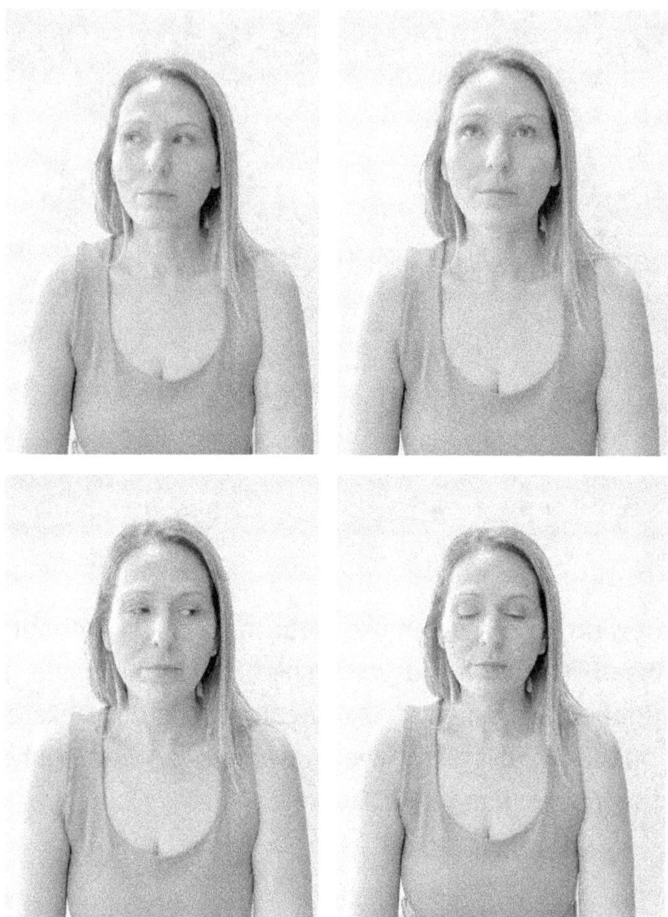

Practise this eye movement just like picturing a clock. Without wrinkling your forehead, start moving your eyes to the left (quarter to) and then to the top (o'clock) as you inhale. As you exhale, rotate your eyes to the right (quarter past) and down (half past). You can practise as per your convenience, in either full, slow or continuous circles, or with a short pause between the moves.

**Benefits:** Improves and coordinates the activities of all the eye muscles to reduce dryness in your eyes and fatigue. It also reduces the redness of the eyes.

# Exercise 14: Gazing at the tip of the nose or Nasikagra Drishti

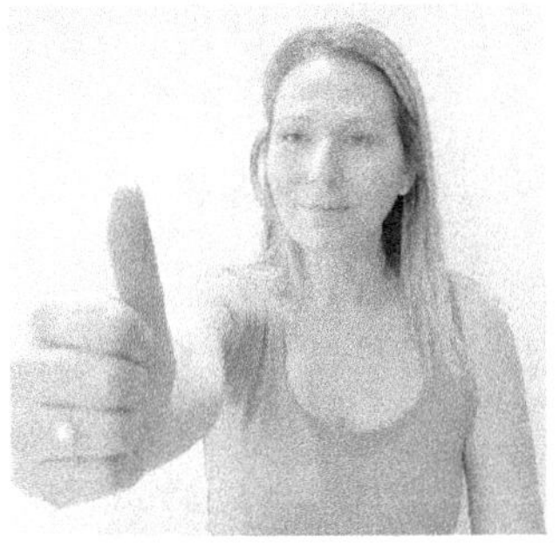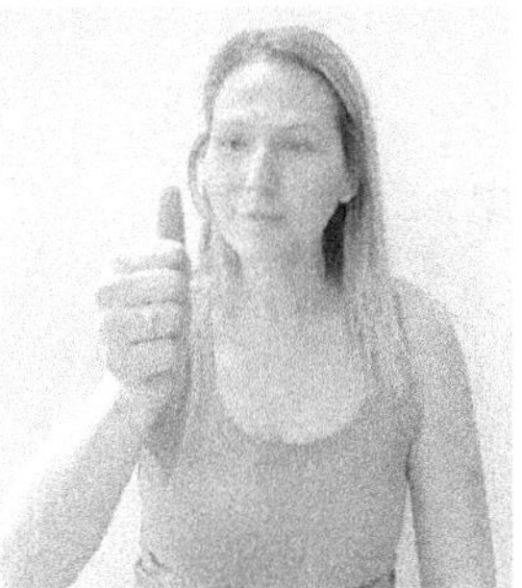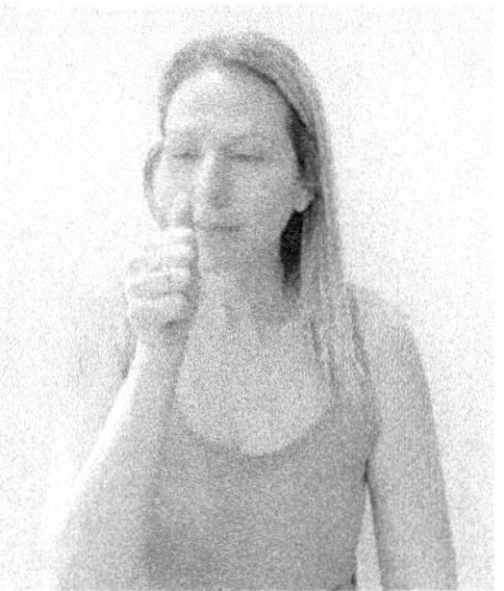

Sit in a comfortable seated position (cross-legged or with legs outstretched). Stretch your left arm in front of your nose. Make a fist with the thumb up and focus both eyes on the tip of the thumb. Inhale as you draw the thumb towards your nose with slow and steady movement, while the eyes focus on and follow the tip of the thumb. Stay for a few seconds with the thumb held at the tip of the nose and the eyes focused on the tip of the thumb. Exhale and slowly stretch your arm out with the eyes focused and following the movement of the tip of the thumb. This equals 1 round. Practise 5-10 times with each hand.

**Benefits:** Improves focus and coordination of eye muscles.

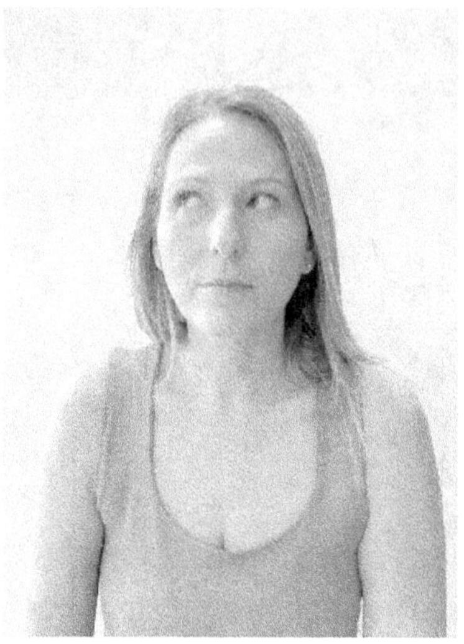 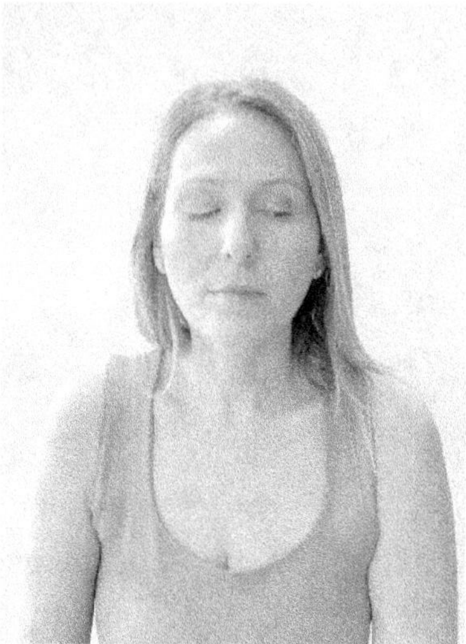

Sit in any comfortable position and lift both your eyes to the top right corner of your vision as you inhale. As you exhale, lower both eyes to the lower left corner. Repeat 5-10 times per side.

**Benefits:** Releases tension from the eye muscles, and prevents and corrects squint.

# Exercise 16:   Toning of bags under the eyes

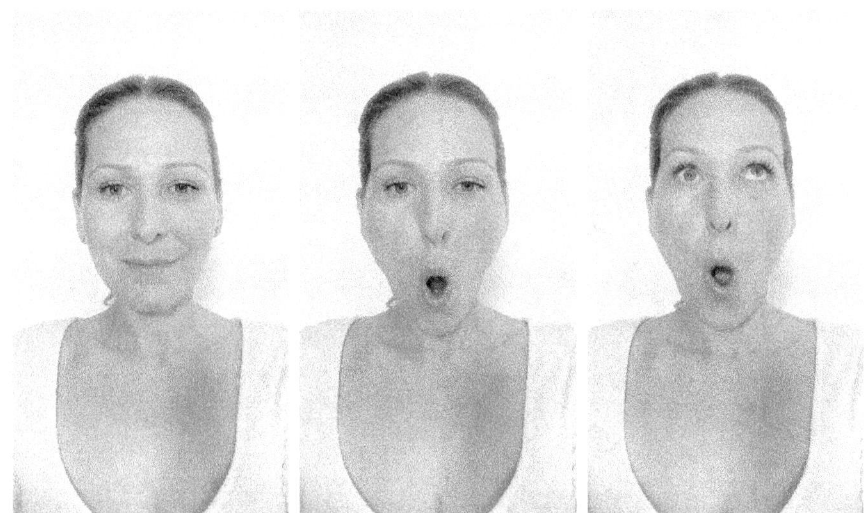

While looking straight ahead, relax your forehead and practise the vowel O. Gaze at the sky and try to tighten your visual focus for as long as you can. Close your eyes and relax your face. Repeat 5-10 times.

**Benefits:** Helps engage all the eye muscles and assists with puffiness and bags under the eyes.

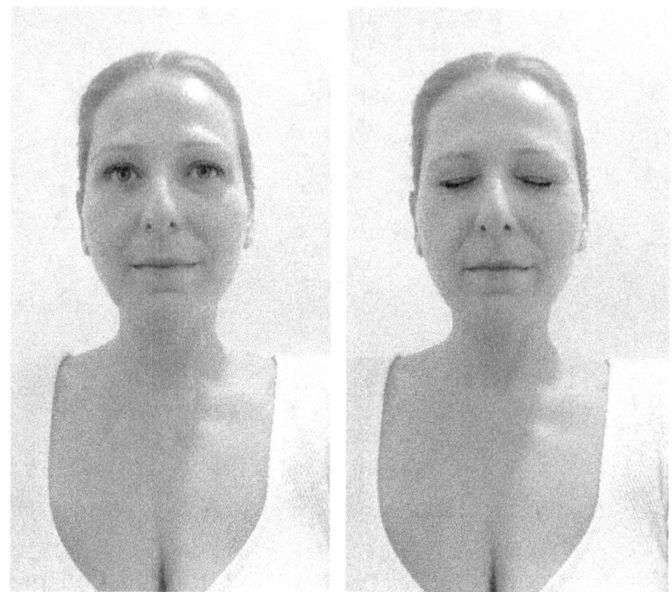

Squeeze your eyes and release. Inhale to squeeze and stay for 5 seconds. Exhale to release and keep your eyes wide open. Practise a minimum of 20 times.

**Benefits:** Engagement of all eye muscles. Can help with the puffiness of eyes and bags under them.

# Exercise 18:   Symmetrical eyebrows

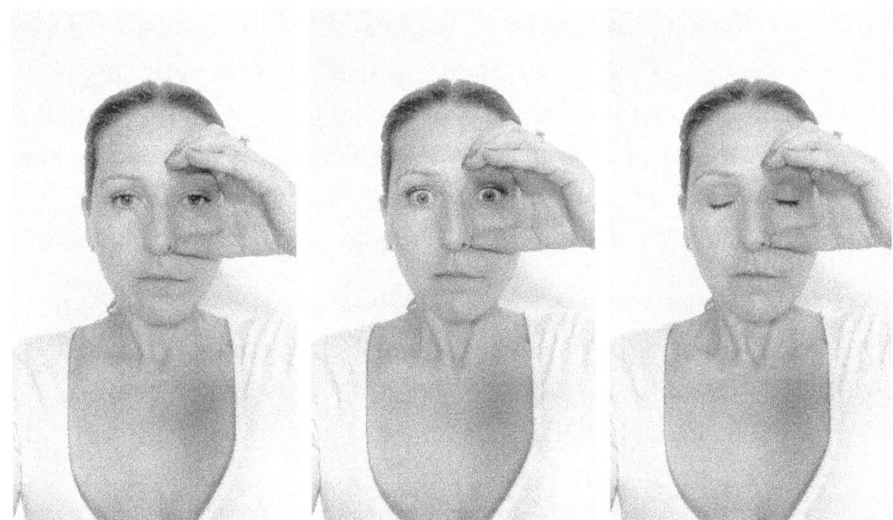

You can practise this exercise only if one of your eyebrows is higher than the other. Otherwise, practice the binocular pose.

If your right eyebrow is higher than the left, then you will exercise to lift your left eyebrow. During the practice, stabilize your right eye with your right hand.

Mould your right hand into a 'C' shape and position the index finger just on top of the eyebrow while the tip of the thumb is positioned beside the nostril.

Open your left eye wide and lift the left eyebrow as high as you can. At the same time, press the fingers of your right hand firmly downwards and sideways so that the right side of the forehead remains still. Hold this position for 10 seconds. Maintain the position, close your eyes and relax for 3 seconds. Repeat 5-10 times.

**Benefits:** Makes the areas around the eyes symmetrical, particularly the eyebrows.

Nasolabial folds, also known as 'smiling lines' can appear even during your early twenties. They run along the sides of the mouth and on the inner side of the cheeks. Excess fat or sagging from sudden weight loss or ageing may result in more visible nasolabial folds that sometimes can reach the corners of the mouth. With the following exercises, lift your cheek muscles to smoothen and reduce these nasolabial folds.

Also, consider that not everyone looks the same and all the face types need exercise as well. However, amongst the various facial shapes, two categories persist—skinny or fuller cheeks. In this chapter, you will find exercises that you can choose as per your needs.

**Option A:**

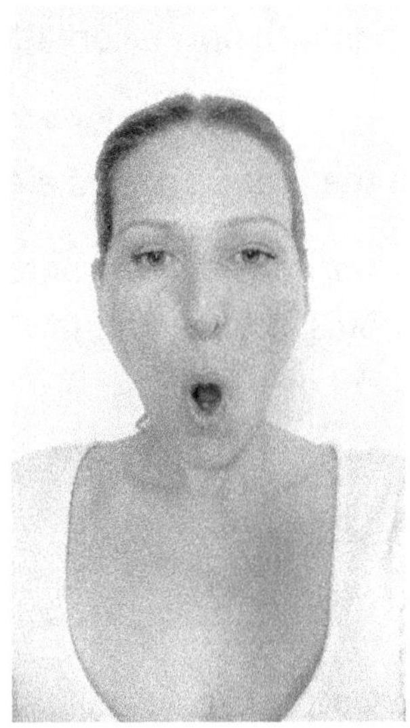

Open your mouth, drop your chin to an 'O' shape and press your upper lip against your teeth to create a more theatrical face. Hold the position for 10 seconds with normal breathing. Repeat 5-10 times.

**Option B:**

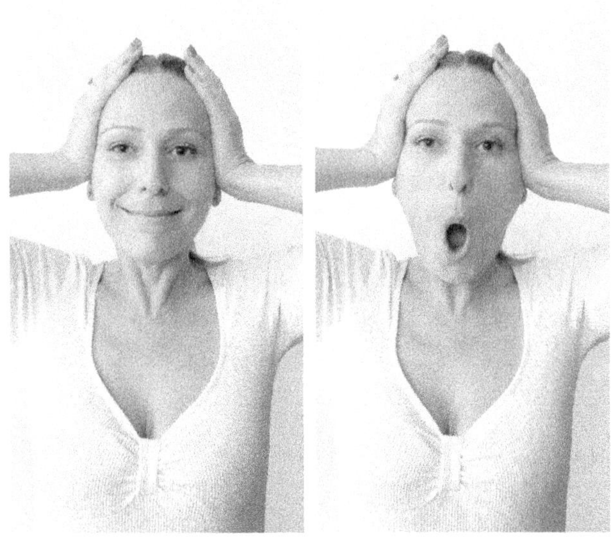

Smile with your palms on your temples. Push in the direction of your ears to lift the sides of your face. Open your mouth, drop your jaw and make an 'O' shape by pressing the upper lip against your teeth. Hold the position for 10 seconds with normal breathing. Repeat 5-10 times.

**Modification:** You can gaze towards the sky if you like to reduce puffiness and smoothen the areas under the eyes.

**Benefits:** Lifts the upper portions and the lines on the side of the face. Reduces the nasolabial folds, shapes the jawline and increases blood flow to your entire face and neck.

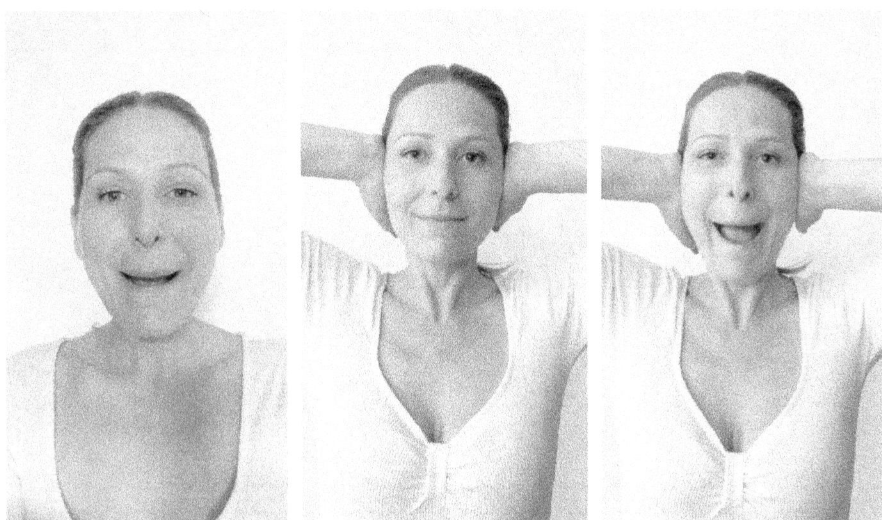

Round your lips over your teeth to lift the corners of your mouth. With your palms over your ears stretch your face towards the back of your head. Open your mouth slightly, round your lips over your teeth and lift the corners of your mouth. Make the 'E' sound to help you focus on the exercise. Hold the position for 10 seconds with normal breathing. Repeat 5-10 times.

**Benefits:** Lifts the lines on the lower face, the corners of the mouth and the cheeks and reduces nasolabial folds.

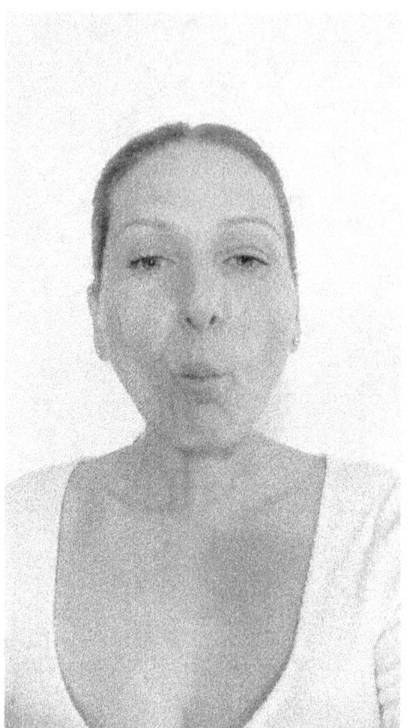

Pull your cheeks in by sucking them in between your teeth. Hold the position for 5 seconds with normal breathing. Release and repeat 10 times.

**Benefits:** Slims the cheeks down and smoothens the nasolabial folds.

**Note:** If there is more fat on the cheeks or if you feel your cheeks are hanging down, you may add more repetitions, or practise this exercise more frequently even during the day. If you feel your cheeks are just right for you, practice the following exercise, the kiss, to benefit.

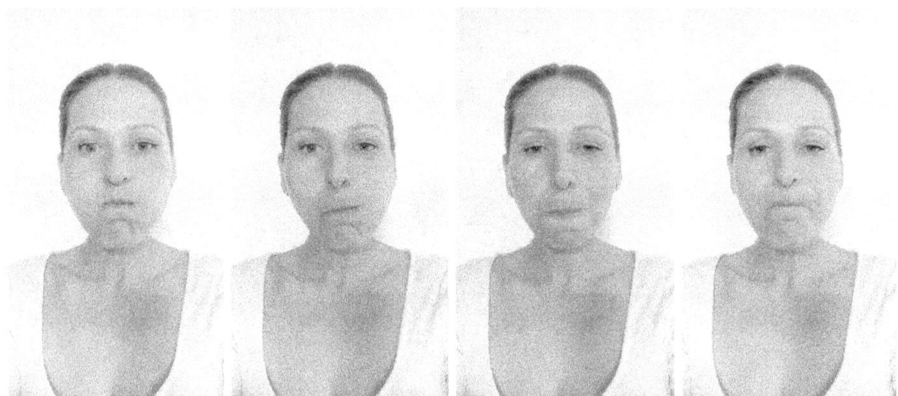

Close your lips and fill your mouth with air while breathing normally. Move the air all around your mouth (right, left, towards the centre of your lips, top of the lips, lower lips and to the sides) while holding the position each time for 5 seconds. Open your mouth to release the pose and relax for 2-3 breaths. Repeat 5-10 times.

**Benefits:** Reduces nasolabial folds and vertical lines on the upper lip. Smoothens the skin around the cheeks and lips.

**Precautions:** Don't practise this exercise if you are suffering from high blood pressure, eye pressure or cardiovascular conditions.

## Exercise 23:  Balloon pose 2 fingers stop

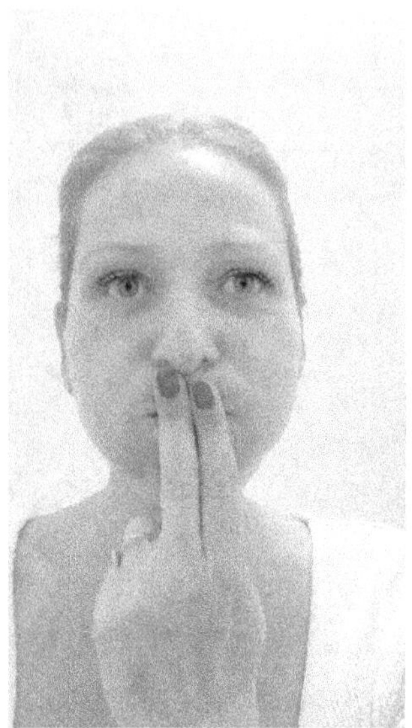

While breathing normally, close your lips to fill your mouth with air and press the pointer and middle finger together on the centre of the lips. The pressing should be gentle but firm enough to feel the pressure inside the cheeks. Hold the position for 5 seconds. Remove your fingers from your lips to open your mouth and release the pose. Relax for 2-3 breaths. Repeat 5-10 times.

**Benefits:** Stimulates the cells and muscles of the inner cheeks. Increases blood circulation and ventilation to the mouth. This practice oxygenates the air in the mouth which helps with oral health and odour.

**Precautions:** Do not practise if you are suffering from high blood pressure, eye pressure or cardiovascular conditions.

**Note:** The excess pressure applied with the 2 fingers may give you a 'happy burning' sensation afterwards. Drink some water between the sessions to combat that sensation.

# Exercise 24:   Tongue rotation on the cheeks

## Option A

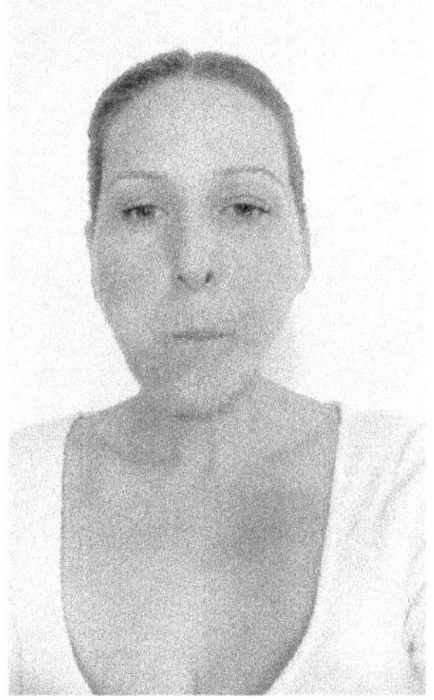

Close your lips, breathe normally and push the right side of your mouth with your tongue. Rotate your tongue slowly 5 times clockwise and 5 times anticlockwise. Repeat the same with the left side of your mouth. Open your mouth to return to a neutral position and relax for 2-3 breaths. Repeat 5-10 times.

## Option B

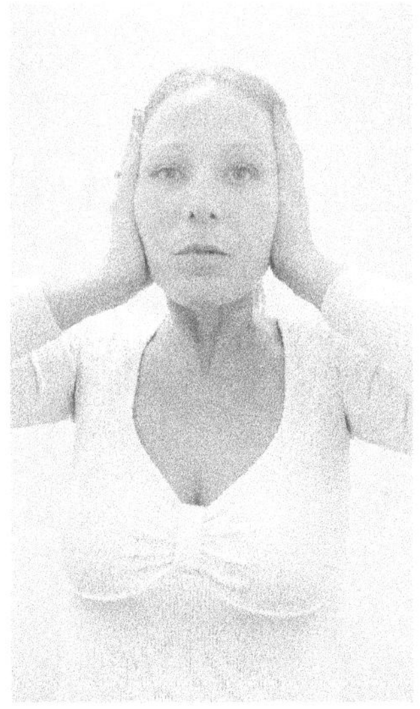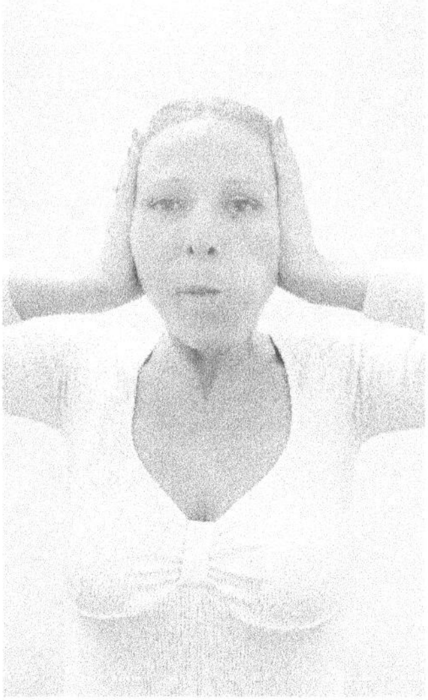

Place your hands on the sides of your face with the thumbs under the ears and the rest of the fingers facing up. Adjust your shoulders comfortably. Practise the same as option A. Release your arms, open your mouth and return to a neutral face while relaxing for 2-3 breaths. Repeat 5-10 times.

**Benefits:** Tones the area around the mouth. Smoothens the nasolabial folds. The stretching of the hands lifts the sides of the face.

# Exercise 25:   Slimmer cheeks

## Option A

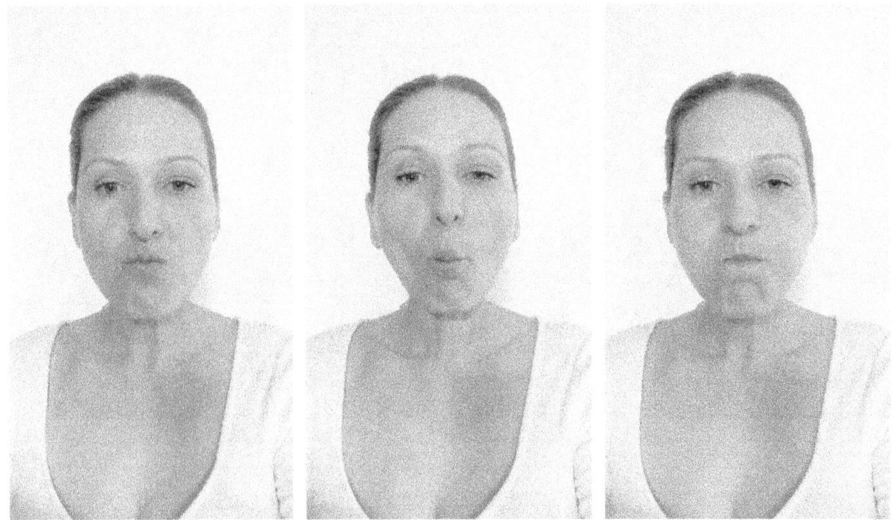

**Kiss:** Bring your cheeks closer to your teeth to make a firm kiss-like shape. Keep breathing normally throughout the whole practice. Keep your eyes wide open and practise the kissing gesture 10 times.

**Fish:** Close your lips and take your cheeks in by sucking them in between your teeth. Hold the position for 5 seconds while breathing normally. Release and repeat 10 times.

**Balloon:** Close your lips to fill your mouth with air while breathing normally. Bring the air toward the centre of your lips and hold for 5 seconds. Open your mouth to release the pose and relax for 2-3 breaths. Repeat 5-10 times.

**Smile:** Smile to release the tension in your facial muscles from the practice.

Repeat 2 times.

**Option B**

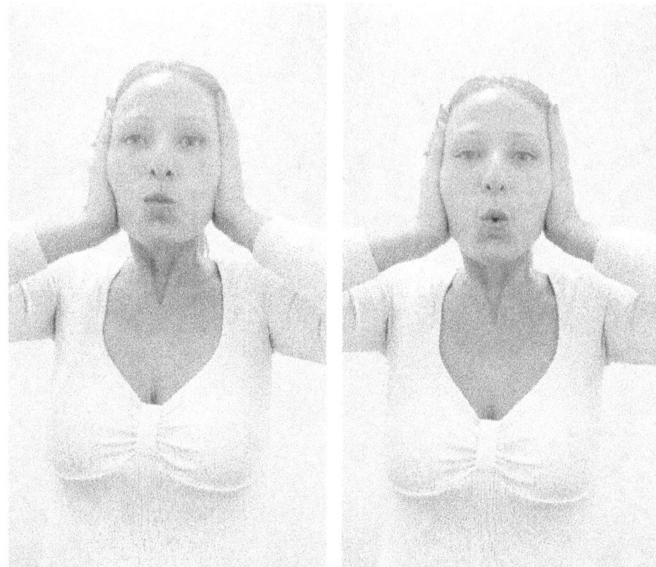

Place your thumbs under your ears and the rest of the fingers facing up on the sides of your face. Stretch your skin towards your ears and upwards. Practise the steps shown in Option A. Blow through your lips 2-3 times before releasing. Repeat 5-10 times.

**Benefits:** Same as Kiss, Fish, Balloon and Smile exercises. Slims the cheeks. Reduces the nasolabial folds. Hand engagement is better for lifting sagging skin.

**Note:** Keep your face and shoulders relaxed during the hand engagement practice.

# Exercise 26:   Cheeks relaxation

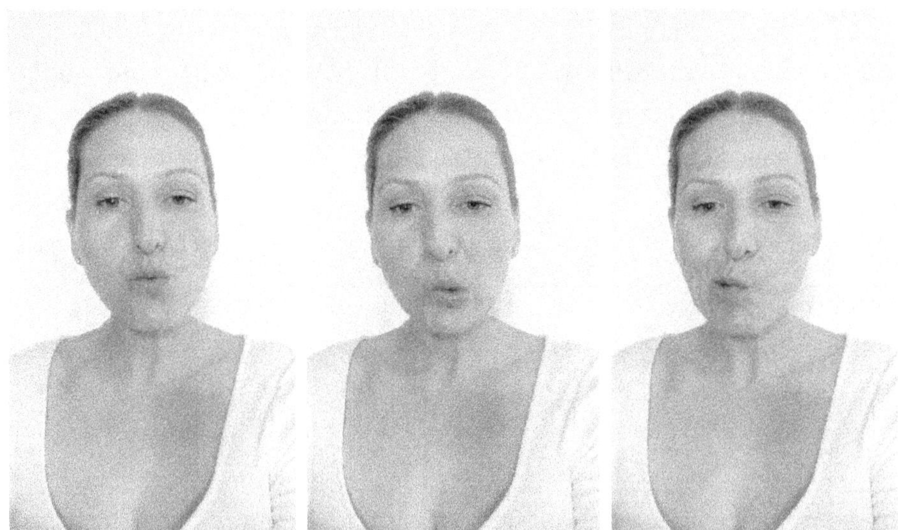

Relax your face and jaw, kiss and move your mouth to the right and hold for 5 seconds. Move your mouth to the left and hold for 5 seconds. Repeat 5-10 times.

**Benefits:** Relaxes the cheek area, slims down the cheeks and reduces the nasolabial folds.

**Option A**

Curl and pull your lips over your teeth, keeping your mouth open. Smile slightly to lift the corners of your mouth. Hold the position for 10 seconds. Repeat 5-10 times.

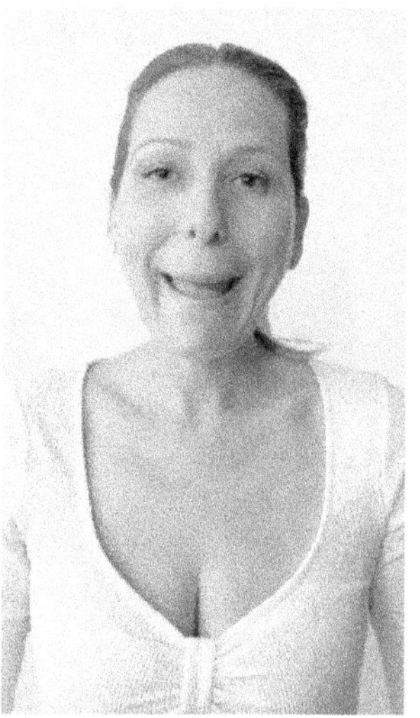

**Option B**

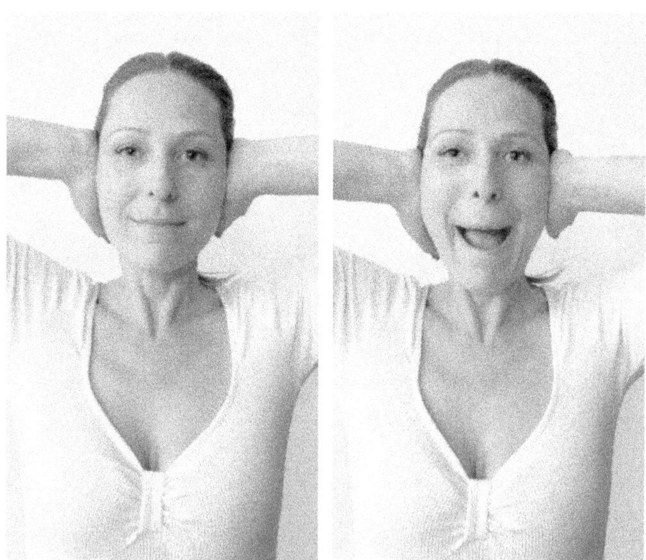

Place the palms of your hands on your ears with the fingers rounded on the back of the head. Curl and pull your lips over your teeth, keeping your mouth open. Smile slightly to lift the corners of your mouth. Hold the position for 10 seconds. Repeat 5-10 times.

**Benefits:** Tones the cheeks, and lifts the corners of the mouth and the lower lines on the face. It also smoothens the nasolabial folds.

**Option A**

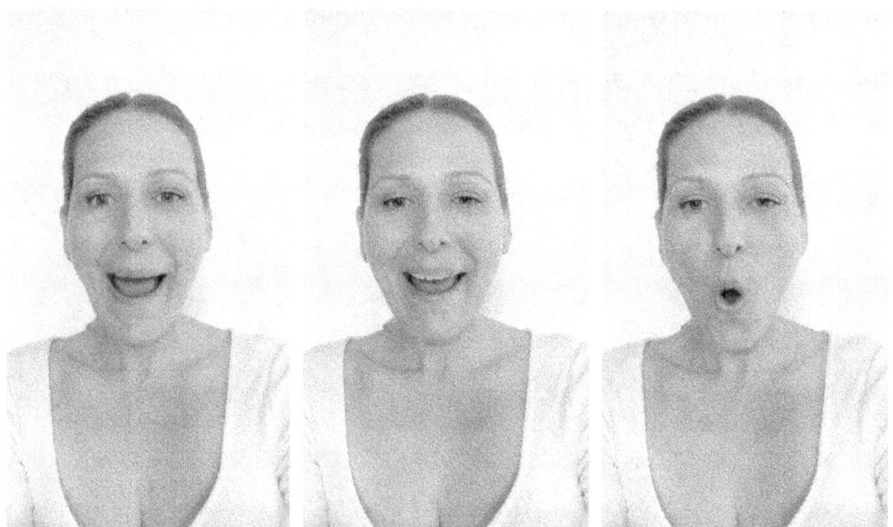

Open your mouth slightly and extend your lower lip over your lower teeth to stretch your mouth. Keep your eyes wide open and your forehead relaxed. Tilt your chin forward and maintain the position for 10 seconds. To come out of the position, practise the vowel O to relax the area around the mouth. Repeat 5-10 times.

**Option B**

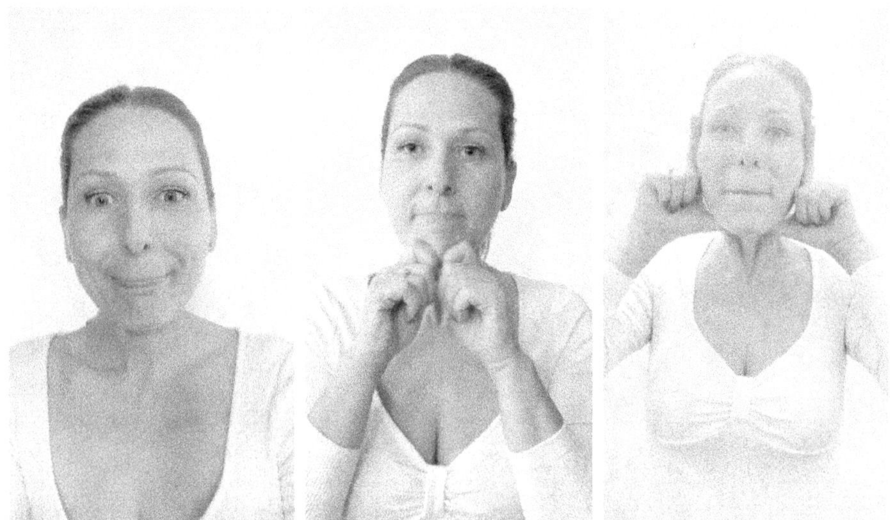

Tilt your chin slightly and bring your lower lip over your top lip and smile. While smiling, make sure the corners of your mouth are at the same level to feel equal tension on both cheeks. To tone the neck area, push your tongue towards the roof of your mouth to engage the neck muscles. Keep your eyes wide open and your forehead relaxed. Place your thumbs under your chin, and your index and middle fingers towards the top of your ears. Adjust the fingers so that you can gently stretch the nasolabial folds. Maintain the position for 10 seconds. To come out of the position, practise the vowel O to relax the area around the mouth. Repeat 5-10 times.

**Benefits:** Increases blood circulation to the face and neck, tones the bags under the eyes, smoothens the nasolabial folds, and lifts the cheeks and the corners of the mouth. It also defines and makes the cheeks look fuller.

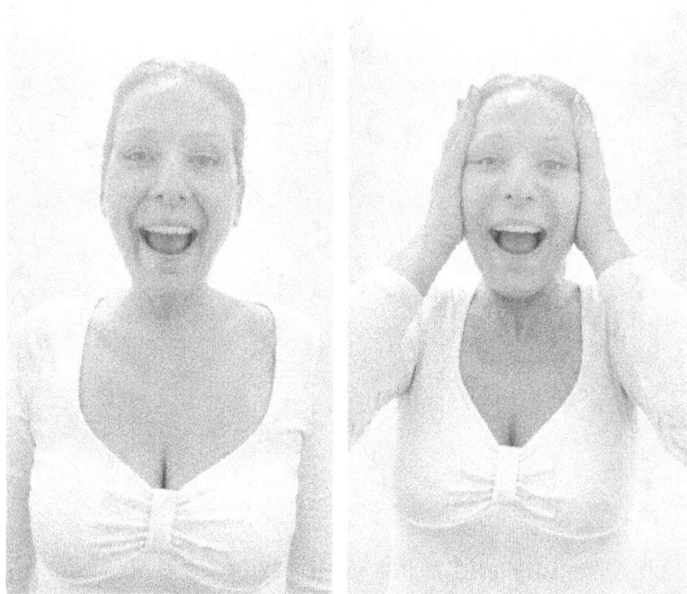

Open your mouth and extend your lower lip over your lower teeth to stretch your mouth. Keep your eyes wide open with your forehead relaxed. Tilt your chin forward slightly and maintain the position for 10 seconds.

To tone the neck, push your tongue towards the roof of your mouth to engage the neck muscles. Try to keep your eyes wide open and your forehead relaxed. Position your palms on top of the cheeks and slide them toward your ears and up. Maintain the position for 10 seconds. Repeat 5-10 times.

**Benefits:** Tones the bags under the eyes, smoothens the nasolabial folds, lifts the cheeks and the corners of the mouth as well as defines and makes the cheeks look fuller.

By looking at someone's mouth, you can identify their age and their emotions too. When the corners of the mouth are up, we can see that someone is happy! When they are down, we look unhappy. With these exercises, you can work on your mouth and lips to look younger and happier.

As you age, your lips lose their firmness and age lines appear on them too. Your mouth and lips get a lot of exercise every day as you talk, smile, yawn, chew and kiss. However, with these exercises, you can stimulate the muscles in that area to get firmer and smoother lips.

Before and after your practice, remember to apply lip balm to avoid any breakage from the stretching of the lips. If you feel it needs to be reapplied during the practice, please do so. Practise in front of a mirror to check and correct the symmetry of the corners of the mouth and other facial muscles.

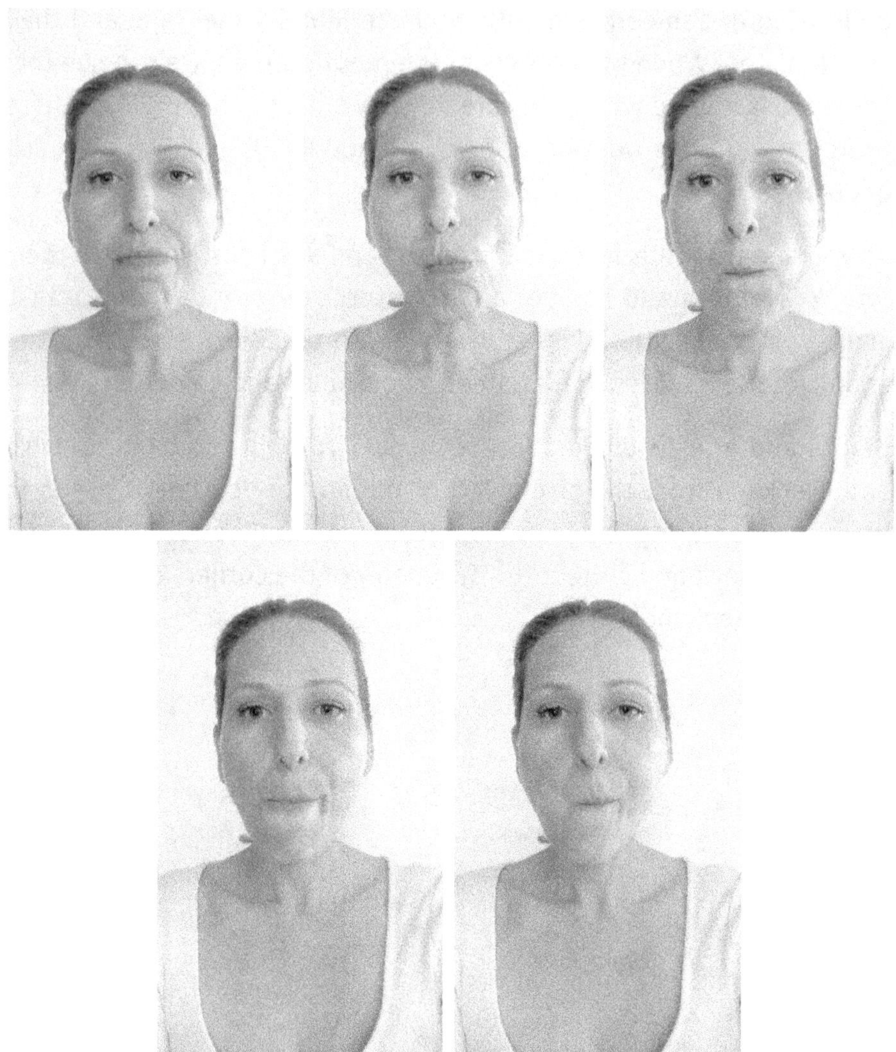

With your mouth closed, rotate your tongue 5 times clockwise and 5 times anticlockwise all around your gums and as far back as possible.

**Benefits:** Smoothens the lines all around the mouth, from the moustache area to the sides of the lips and upper chin, including the nasolabial folds.

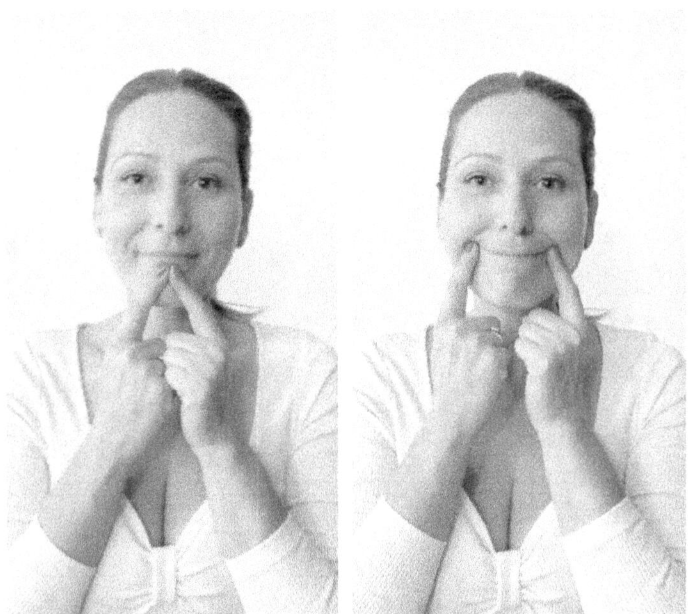

With your mouth closed, smile. Make sure the corners of your mouth are even and at the same level. Maintain the position and place both your index fingers on your chin as you smile. Smile more and with your lips closed or slightly open, slide your index fingers up to the corners of your lips to lift them. You can rest your tongue behind your lower teeth. Stay in that position for 3-5 breaths and release. Repeat 5-10 times.

**Benefits:** Smoothens the lines and wrinkles under the mouth, tones the chin, and lifts the corner of the mouth, creating a younger, happier-looking face.

**Option A**

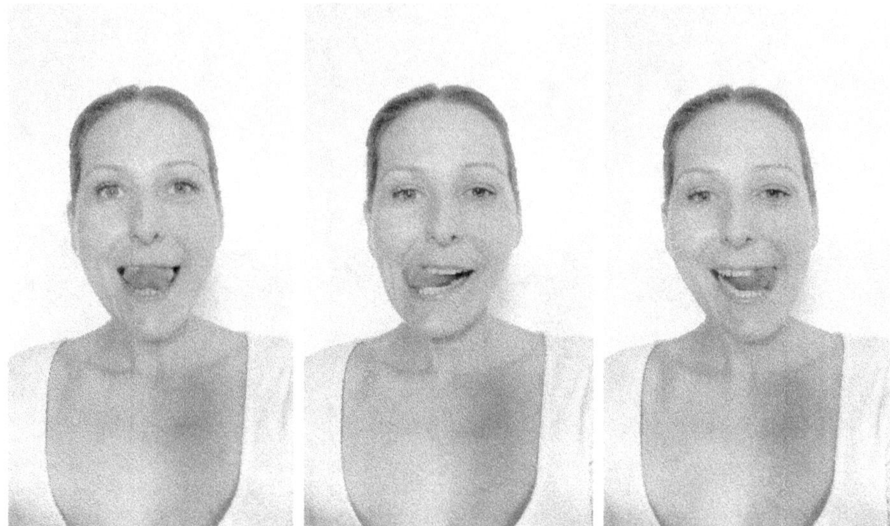

Smile with your mouth open. Ensure that the corners of your mouth are even or at the same level. Bring your tongue out and upwards in an attempt to touch the tip of your nose and hold the smile and the tongue steady for 5 seconds. Maintain the position and slowly move it to the right. Hold the smile and the tongue for 5 seconds. Now, move it slowly to the left and hold for 5 seconds. Return to a neutral position and smile to release any tension in the area around the mouth. Repeat 5-10 times.

**Option B**

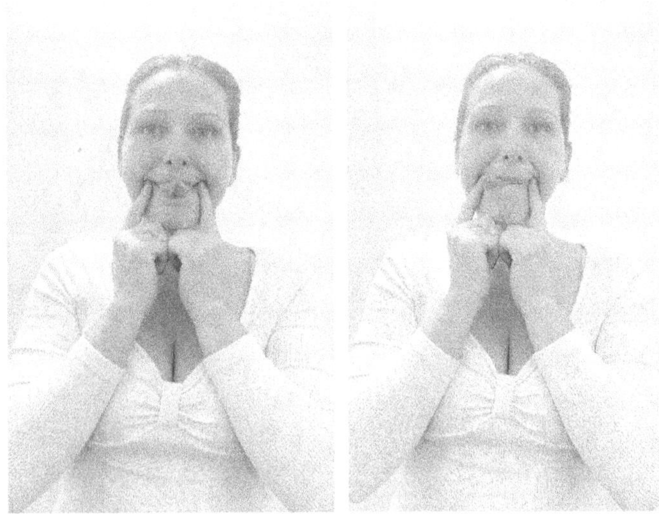

If you want to work harder on lifting your cheeks and mouth, place both your thumbs on your chin and smile. With your index fingers, slowly slide to lift the corners of your mouth. Open your mouth, bring your tongue out and push it up in an attempt to touch the tip of your nose and hold for 5 seconds. Move your tongue to the right and hold for 5 seconds, then move it to the left slowly and hold for 5 seconds. Release it and return to a neutral position and smile to release any tension in the area around the mouth. Repeat 5-10 times.

**Benefits:** Smoothens the lines and wrinkles in the area around the mouth, tones the chin, cheeks and corners of the mouth, creating a younger and happier-looking face.

**Option A**

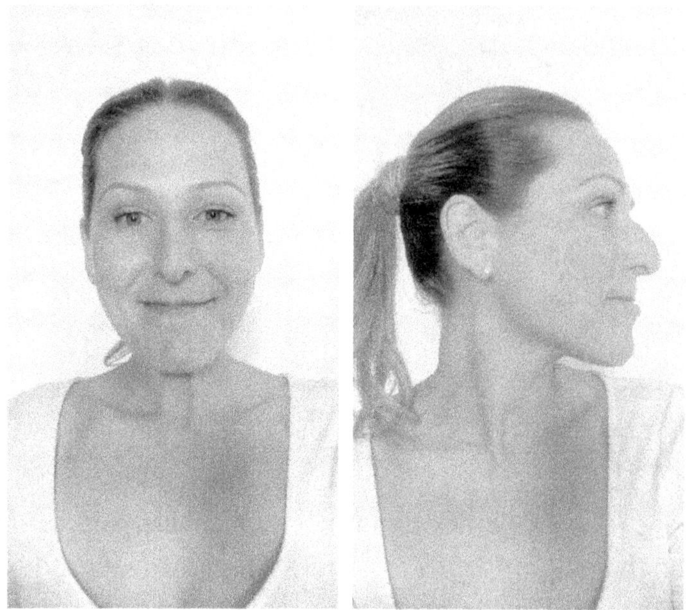

Tilt your chin slightly and bring your lower lips over your top lips and smile. While smiling, make sure the corners of your mouth are even or at the same level. To tone the neck area, push your tongue towards the roof of your mouth to engage the muscles of the neck.

**Option B**

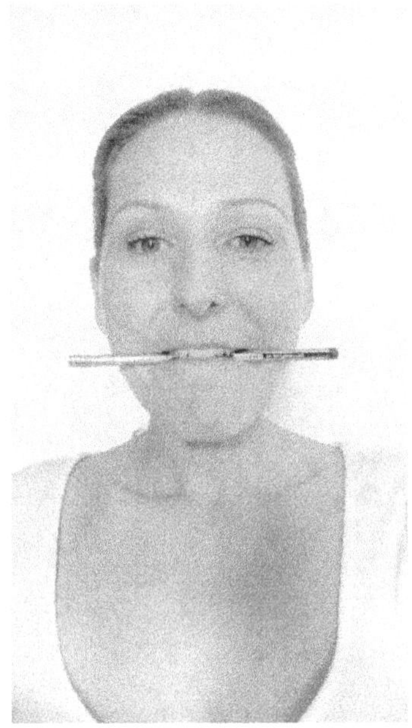

If you want to work harder on lifting your cheeks, you can take a pen or pencil, and place it horizontally close to the corners of your mouth, behind your canine teeth. Relax while holding the pose with normal breathing for 10 seconds and release. Repeat 5 times with 3 seconds of relaxation in between.

**Benefits:** Lifts up the cheeks, neck area and corners of the mouth.

# Exercise 34:   Symmetrical mouth

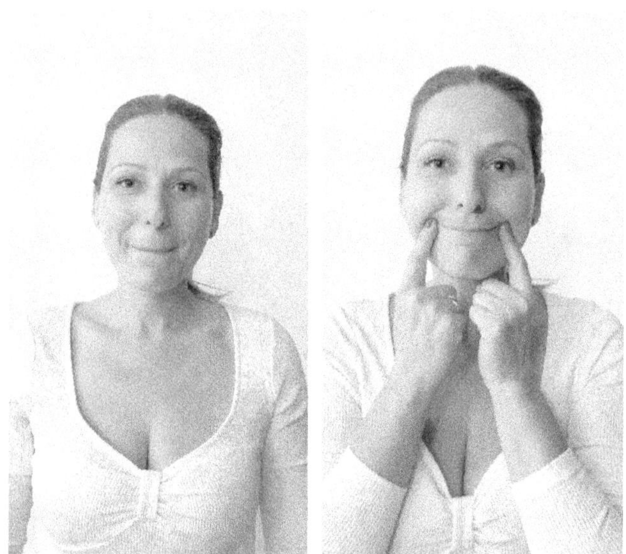

There are people whose smile is not symmetrical. This happens when you chew your food from one side of your mouth, which means you exercise the muscles on this particular side while the opposite side remains idle. Remember to chew your food from both sides of your mouth so they are even.

To practise this exercise, lock your lips over your teeth while looking straight ahead. Place your index fingers on the corners of the mouth and lift them evenly. Fix your gaze towards the sky while maintaining the position of the mouth/fingers. Move your chin up slightly and tilt your head back as per your comfort. Hold the position for 5 seconds. To release the pose, return your chin and head to the neutral position, look straight, remove your fingers, and release the lips. Take a few breaths and repeat the exercise 3-5 times.

**Benefits:** Will make your mouth symmetrical and reduce the lines on your upper lip and nasolabial folds. It also tones your cheeks, neck and double chin while lifting the corners of your mouth to give you a symmetrical smile.

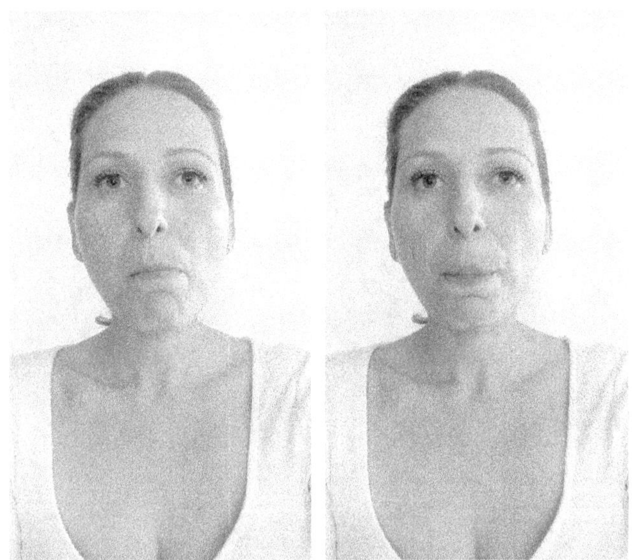

With your mouth closed, rotate your tongue on your inner lips 5 times clockwise and 5 times anticlockwise.

**Benefits:** Smoothens the lines on and around the lips.

**Option A**

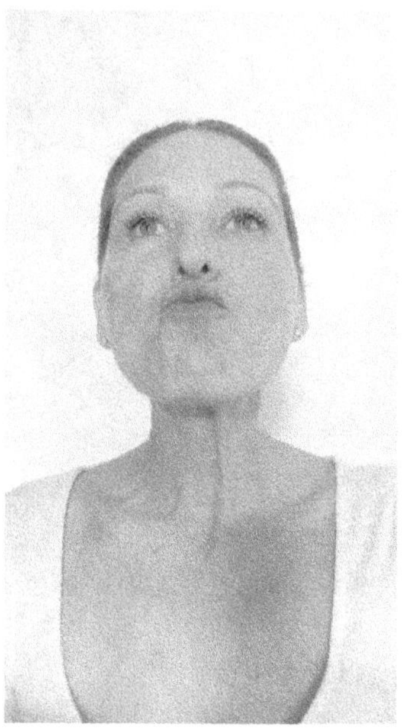

Tilt your chin up and bring your cheeks closer to your teeth to form a firm kiss-like shape. You can close your eyes if you like, and relax your forehead. Repeat 5-10 times.

**Option B**

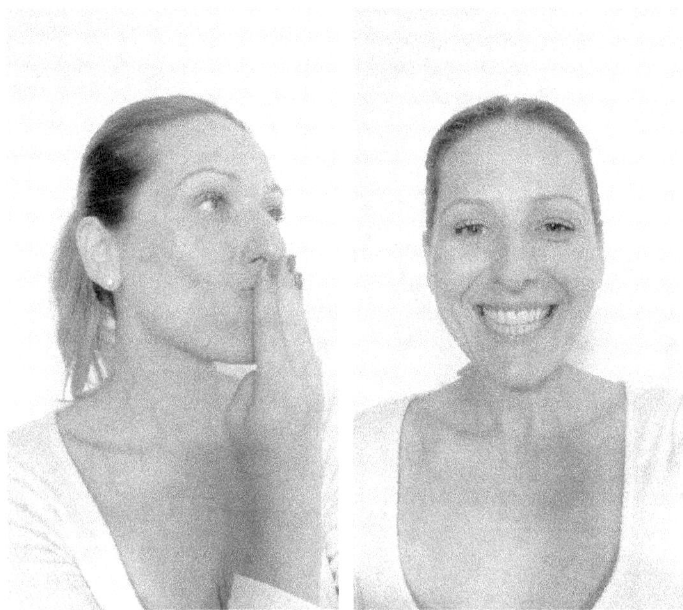

With your head in a neutral position, bring your cheeks closer to your teeth to form a firm kiss-like shape. You can close your eyes if you like and relax your forehead. Place your index, middle and ring finger on your lips and apply pressure, as if you are giving a flying kiss. Repeat 5-10 times. After you have finished, smile to relax the muscles.

**Benefits:** Strengthens and firms the area around the mouth, tones the muscles in the jaw, mouth and cheek areas, gives shape to the lips and gives them a natural rose colour while reducing the nasolabial folds and slimming the cheeks.

**Awareness:** If you believe in the power of the universe, kissing it and sending love to it can attract the same in your life.

## Option A

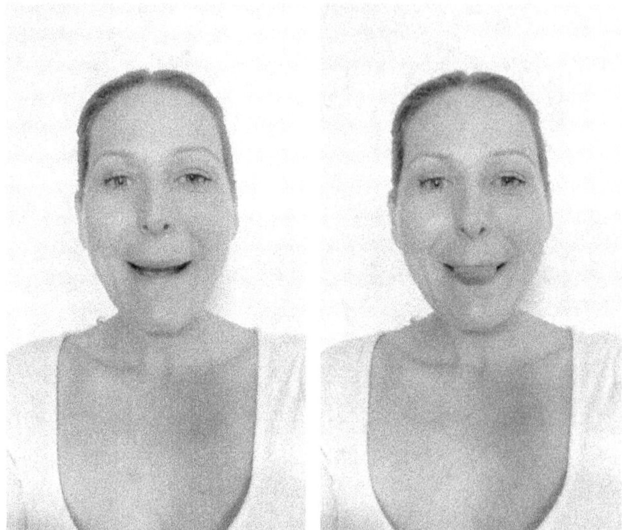

Curl and pull your lips over your teeth, keeping your mouth open. Smile slightly to lift the corners of your mouth. Bring your tongue out, place it between the lips and bite with pressure. Hold the position for 5 seconds and release. Repeat 5-10 times.

## Option B

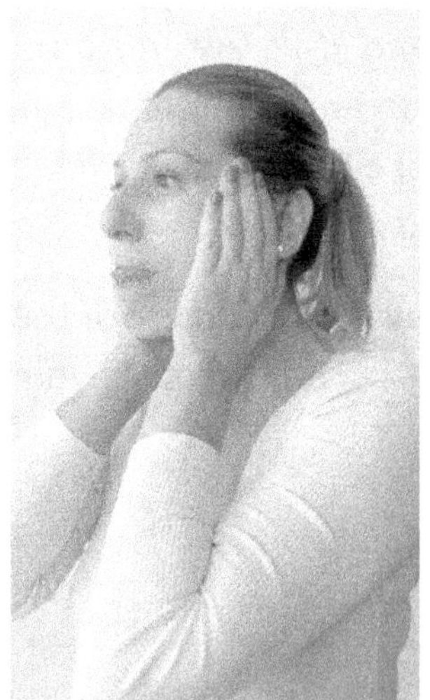

Curl and pull your lips over your teeth, keeping your mouth open. Smile slightly to lift the corners of your mouth. Bring your tongue out, place it between the lips and bite with pressure. Place both hands on the sides of your face and pull towards your ears with firm pressure. Hold the position for 5 seconds and release. Repeat 5-10 times. This is recommended if you want to tone your mouth to soften and reduce wrinkles that usually appear with age.

**Option C**

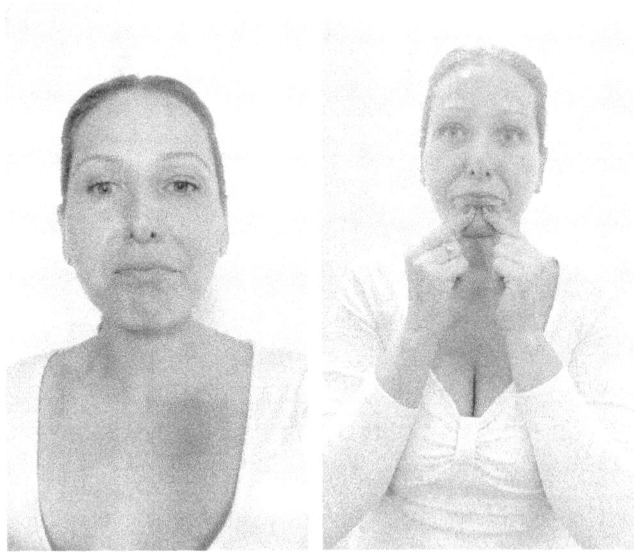

Close your mouth slightly and vibrate your lips to make a humming sound for 10 seconds. Inhale to start the vibration. Exhale as the vibration is in progress. Repeat 5-10 times. Place both thumbs under the chin and index fingers on top of the chin to vibrate your lips for 10 seconds. Release and repeat 5-10 times.

**Benefits:** Smoothens the lines around the mouth and nasolabial folds. Lifts your cheeks and the corners of the mouth and makes the lips fuller.

# Exercise 38:   Weight lifting

## Option A

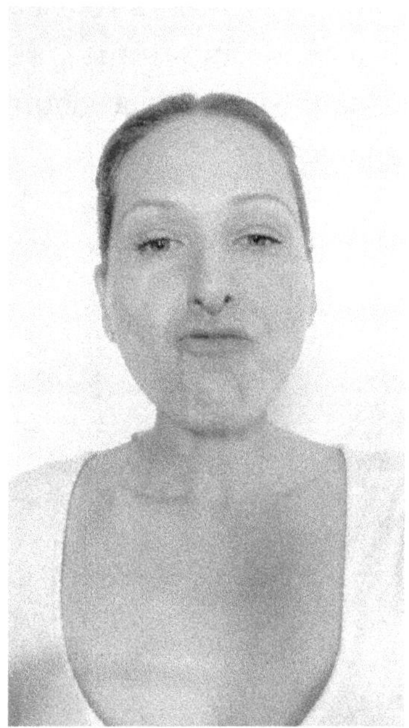

Inhale to lift your chin and purse your lips firmly like a kiss. Remain in the position for a few seconds, and exhale to release and return to the neutral position. Try this for a few days if you are a beginner. Repeat 10 times.

**Option B**

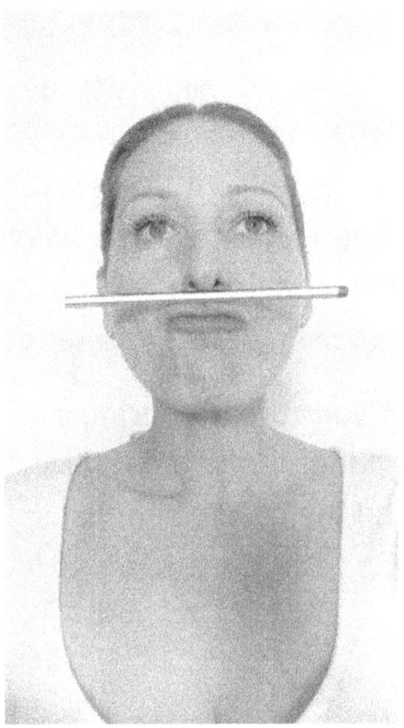

After you have strengthened your lips, you can try placing a wax crayon, a pencil, a marker or a heavier and non-sharpened item on top of your lips. Repeat 10 times.

**Benefits:** This is a weight-lifting exercise for strengthening and toning the lips and the mouth area as well as the cheeks. After 2 months of daily practice, you will be able to see your lips becoming shapely and rosy.

**Counter-pose:** After this exercise, practise the smile to relax the muscles around the mouth.

With this group of exercises, everyone can benefit, regardless of whether they want to work on their face as the neck muscles get stronger and toned while at the same time providing relief from stiffness in the area. During any of these exercises, if you stretch your tongue, it will benefit the muscles at the back of the throat and the sides of the neck. The involvement of the tongue in your practice can increase work on your facial muscles and reduce snoring.

Remember not to hold your breath during these sessions. Instead of normal breathing, be mindful of synchronizing your breath with the movements by following the cues given.

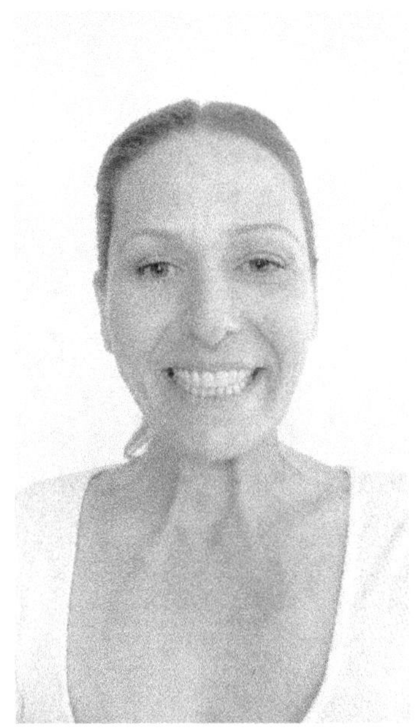

Clench your upper and lower molars together (i.e. your back teeth) and lift your chin slightly. Smile while maintaining the pose to pull your mouth sideways. Engage your jaw to contract the neck muscles. Exhale to return to the neutral position. Repeat 10 times.

**Benefits:** Firms, tones and shapes the neck and the jawline. Lifts the double chin and chest area.

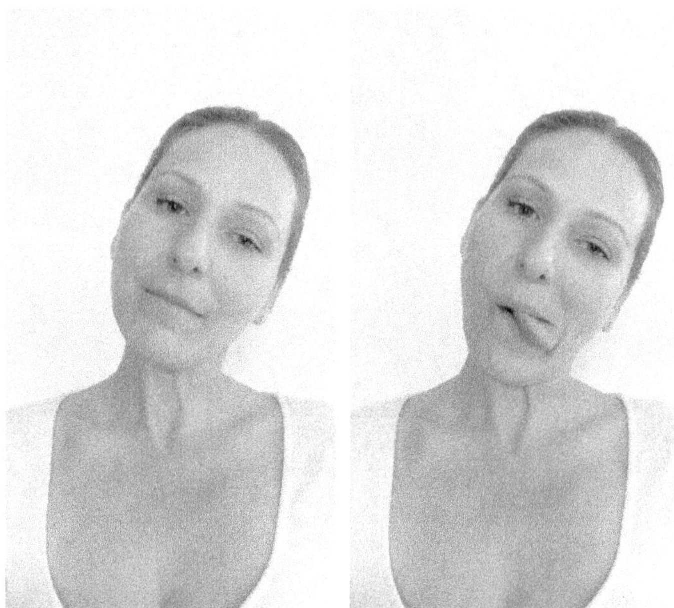

Bend your head to one side toward your shoulder and bring your tongue out as far as possible to the same side. Engage your throat to stimulate the neck muscles. Repeat 10 times.

**Benefits:** Tones and shapes the jawline. Makes the frontal and side areas of the neck firm.

**Precautions:** The tongue exercises should not be practised if you are suffering from face or tongue conditions.

**Note:** For a lesser impact, keep the head straight to tone only the front of the neck and move your tongue slowly from side to side.

**Option A**

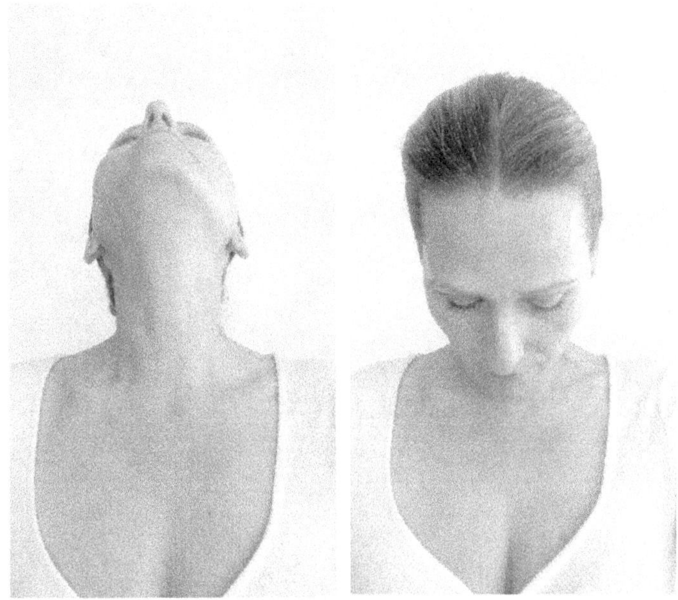

Inhale to move your head up and engage the muscles of the neck. Stay there for 5 seconds. Exhale to move your head from the back of the neck down, in an attempt to touch the chin to chest. Repeat 10 times.

**Option B**

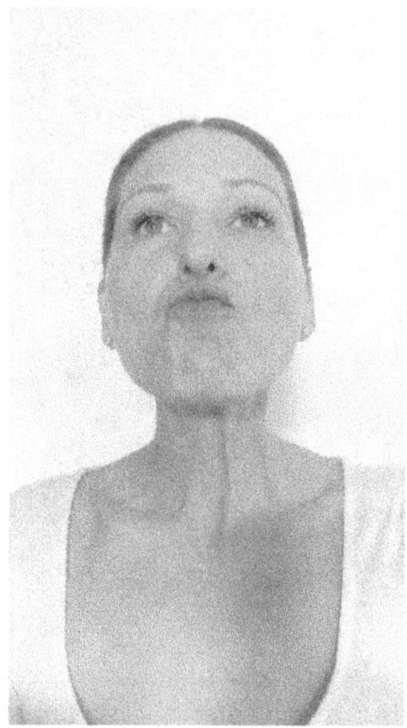

Tilt your head up and practise the fish pose or the kiss exercise to tone the cheeks, lift the double chin and relax the muscles at the back of the neck. Repeat 5-10 times.

**Benefits:** Firms the double chin, slims and tones the cheeks and offers relief from tension in the neck and mid-back region.

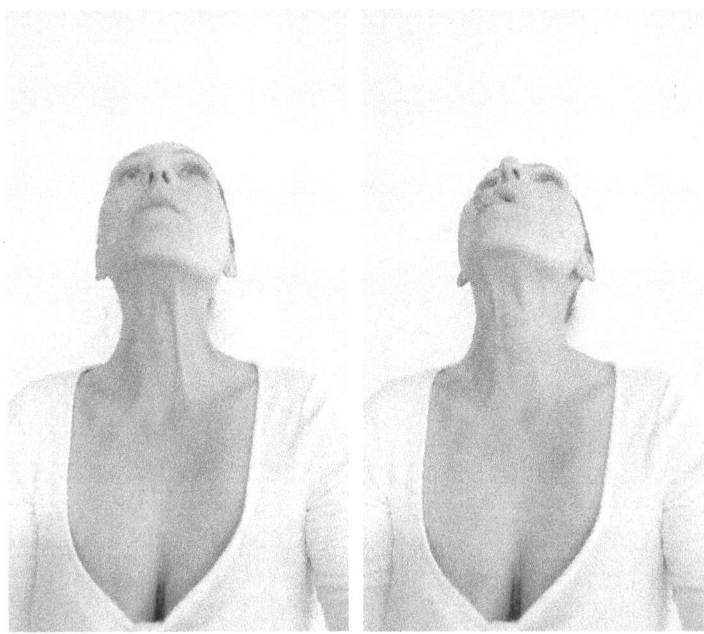

Keep looking straight and move your head up. Bring your tongue out and push it up. Move your tongue slowly to the right and hold it there for 5 seconds. Then slowly move it to the left and hold for 5 seconds. Repeat 5-10 times.

**Benefits:** Strengthens the neck and the jawline, lifts the double chin, slims and tones the cheeks while relaxing the muscles at the back of the neck.

**Option A**

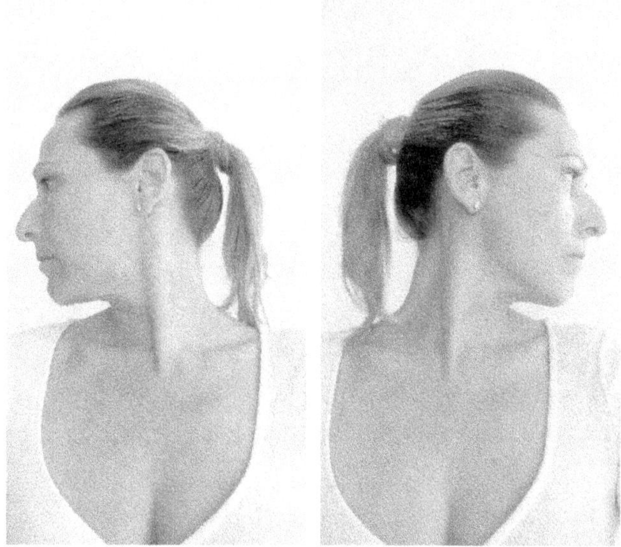

Move your head left-to-right in a continuous motion with normal breathing. Repeat 5-10 times or inhale to turn your head from the neutral position to the left, hold the position for 3-5 seconds and engage your neck muscles. Exhale to come to the centre. Inhale to turn your head to the right, hold the position for 3-5 seconds and engage your neck muscles. Exhale to come to the centre. This is 1 round. Repeat 5-10 rounds.

**Option B**

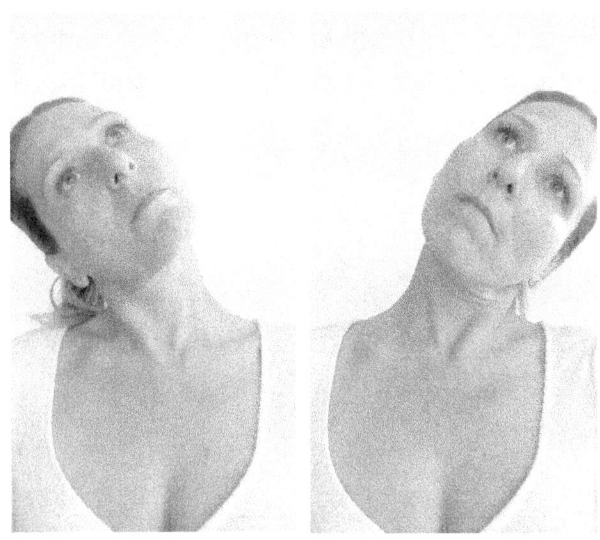

Bend your head from side to side and attempt to keep your ear parallel to your shoulder. To stretch the muscles at the side of the neck more, push the opposite shoulder slightly downward and backwards. Repeat 5-10 times.

**Option C**

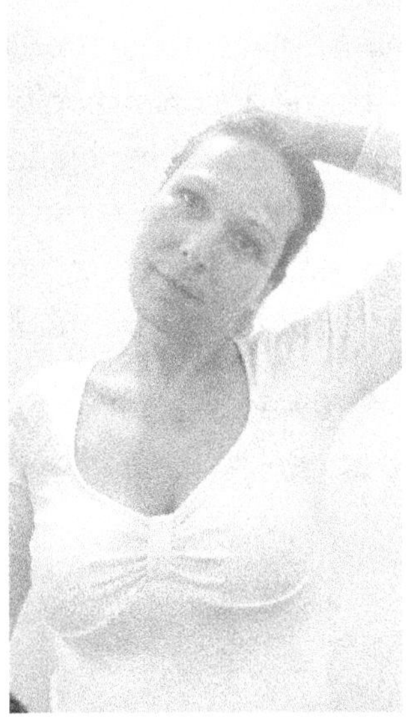

Same as option B. Bend your head to the right and keep your left arm down at the side of your trunk. Lift your right arm over your head to place the fingers on top of the ear. Gently push it to the right and feel the stretch on the left side of the neck and shoulder. Repeat 5-10 times on each side.

**Option D**

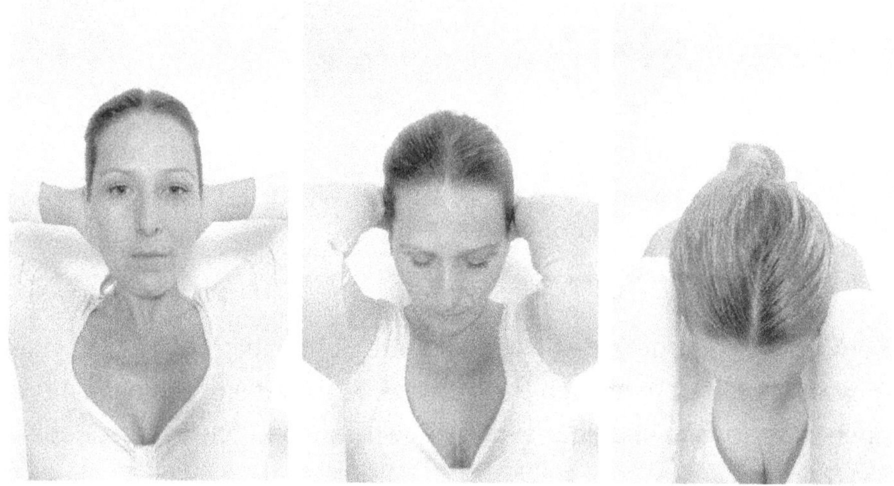

If you feel the need for an extra stretch than just obtained by practising head up and down, interlock your fingers and place them on the back of your head above your hairline. Inhale to lift your head, and open your chest and elbows to maximum capacity to feel the stretch on your mid back, shoulders and shoulder blades. Exhale to move your elbows parallel to your head, bend your head and gently press it down to look at your feet or be parallel to the ground. You should feel the stretch on your neck and upper back. Do not strain. Repeat 5 times.

**Benefits:** Relaxes and stretches the neck muscles. Offers relief from tension in the mid back, upper back, shoulders, and neck areas.

**Option A**

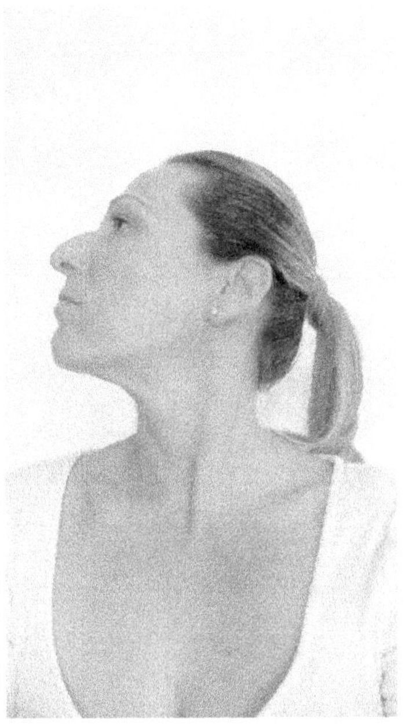

From the neutral position, inhale to turn your head left parallel to your shoulder and lift your head to a 45° angle in that direction. Relax your forehead and stay in position for 5 seconds. Exhale to return to the neutral position. If you are not feeling the stretch, touch the left shoulder with the opposite hand (for example, if you are looking to the left, with the right hand). Repeat the same with the right side to complete 1 round. Repeat 5-10 times.

**Option B**

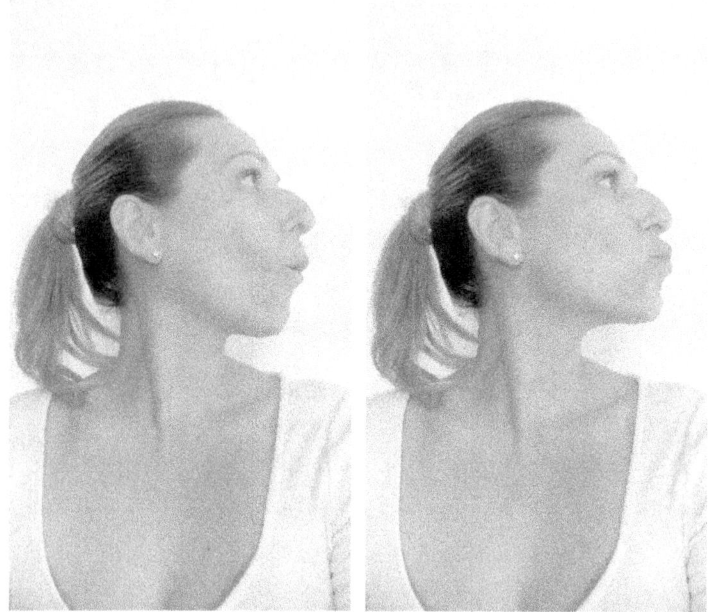

Same as option A but do the fish if you aim to slim down the cheeks or the kiss to tone the cheeks. Repeat 5-10 times.

**Benefits:** Makes the neck and the jawline firm, lifts the double chin, and tones the muscles at the side of the neck. Offers relief from tension in the neck, upper back and shoulders.

# Cooling Down

In every form of exercise, there is a cool-down phase with specific exercises to help your body stretch the tensed muscle and relax. In face yoga, you have worked on the head, face, neck, shoulders and chest areas so far. You can do the upper body stretch exercises and practise tapping at the end in the manner described below.

If you are seated in a cross-legged position, then you need to cool down your back as well as your legs. Try the following:

- Dynamic back stretch pose or roll-up or Gatyatmak Paschimottanasana

- Back stretching pose or forward bend or Paschimottasana

- Child's pose or Shashankasana

If you are standing during your practice, try to cool down your body with:

- Hand-to-foot pose or Padahastasana

- Standing head between knees pose or Utthita Janu Sirshasana

- Mountain pose or downward dog or Adho Mukha Svanasana

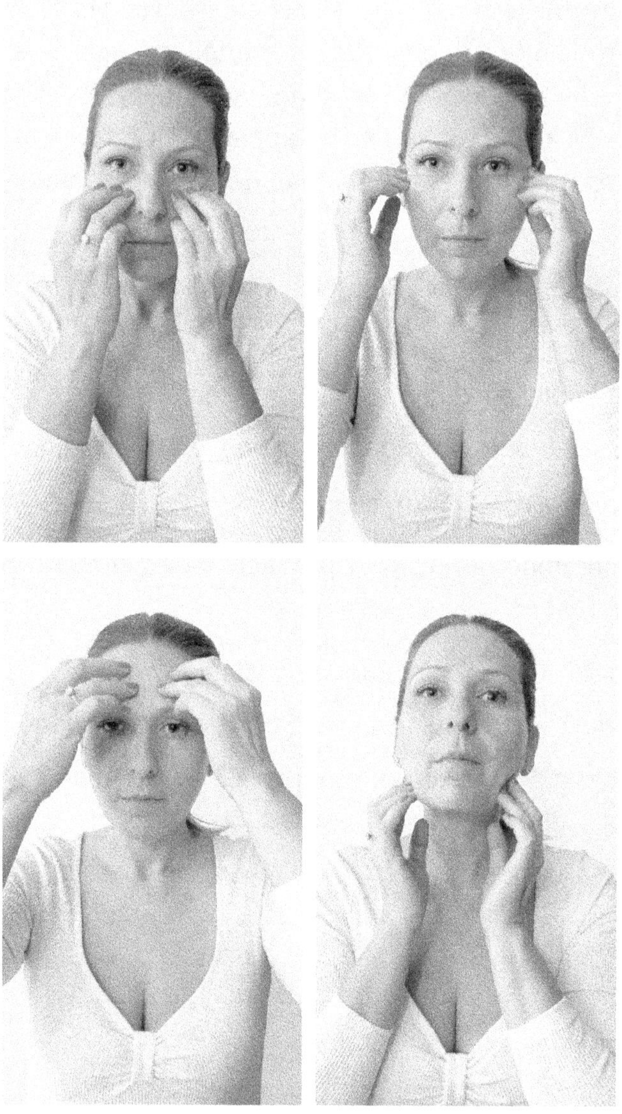

Tapping can be done at any point during the day, especially if you want to increase your focus or relax. It can be done to cool the muscles down after practising exercises. After the face massage, you can choose to do a full face tapping or slapping.

With your middle fingers start tapping the:

- Top of your head for 10 seconds
- Sides of your head and temples for 10 seconds
- Back of your head for 10 seconds
- Forehead in a vertical and horizontal direction for 10 seconds
- Eyebrows from the centre to the sides for 10 seconds
- Under the eyes for 10 seconds
- Around the eyeballs for 10 seconds in a circular movement
- The nose (sides and under) for 10 seconds
- Cheekbones for 10 seconds
- Rest of the cheek for 10 seconds
- Jawline for 10 seconds
- Front of the neck for 10 seconds
- Sides of the neck for 10 seconds
- Back of the neck for 10 seconds

**Benefits:** It calms you mentally. It also removes toxins and reduces puffiness since it encourages the flow of lymph back into the bloodstream via the lymph nodes. It improves the flow of oxygen to the skin, plumps the face and smoothens wrinkles by stimulating collagen production and normalizing the activity of oil and sweat glands.

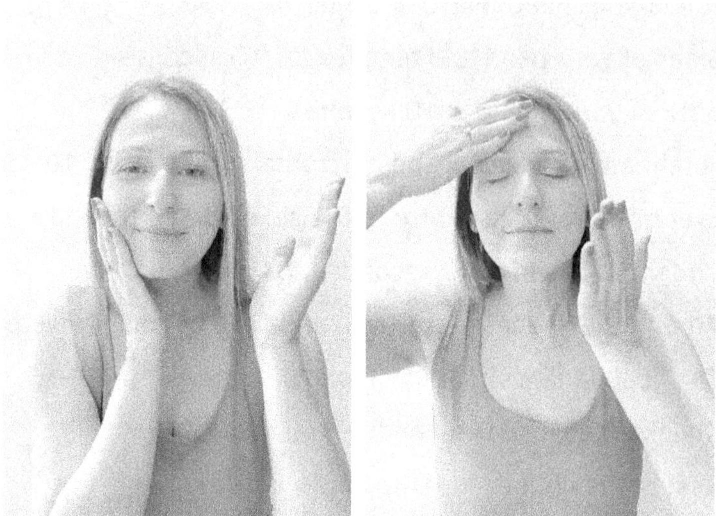

Slapping is an alternative cooling-down technique. You can either choose to do tapping first and then slapping, or either of them alone.

Gently slap your face with your fingers in a way similar to tapping. Beware of the area around your eyes when slapping. Try to avoid this area since it can lead to you hitting some ocular muscles or the eyes themselves.

**Benefits:** Same as tapping.

# Practising Asanas

While practising face yoga, you may believe that you are working on the face alone but that is not true at all! During this practice, the posture of your body, i.e. whether you are in a seated or standing position, involves your upper body as well. The positioning of the hands which should mostly be bent at the elbows and open sideways at the shoulders, strengthens your chest, shoulders, shoulder blades, upper back, and middle back and if during the practice you are mindful about engaging the core and buttocks you can strengthen these areas as well. To avoid any stiffness in your body, it is recommended that you do some warm-up exercises before your practice and cool down after it.

Face yoga is not limited to face exercises alone, wether we engage the hands or only the facial muscles or with the engagement with only the facial muscles. In the chapter on asanas below, I will give you a selection of poses that most people can practise with ease. In addition to their many benefits, these asanas also benefit our skin and face. Asanas that are chest openers promote more oxygen flow in our body whereas inverted asanas promote better blood circulation to the head and face. Hence, your skin will become healthier, shinier and rosier.

**Exercise 47:    Pelvic Rotation**

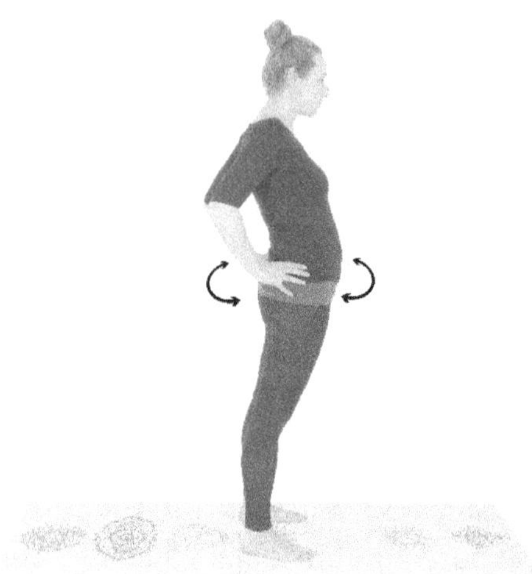

Stand with your feet slightly apart and your spine erect. Place the palms of your hands on top of the hips or the waist and start rotating the pelvis in a slow and controlled circle (360°). Inhale while rotating the pelvis backwards and to the side. Exhale while rotating the pelvis forward and to the centre. A full circle is 1 round. Repeat 5-8 rounds clockwise and anti-clockwise.

**Modification:** For those with severe back pain or imbalance while in this position, practise half rotation to the back for 5-8 rounds and an equal number of rounds towards the front.

**Benefits:** Alleviates pain and reduces stiffness in the lower back, stretches the back muscles and strengthens the abdominal and buttock muscles.

**Awareness:** Sacral (Swadhisthana) Chakra

**Note:** Do a warm-up and cooling-down exercise in between and at the end of the practice.

# Exercise 48:   Full Butterfly or Poorna Titali Asana

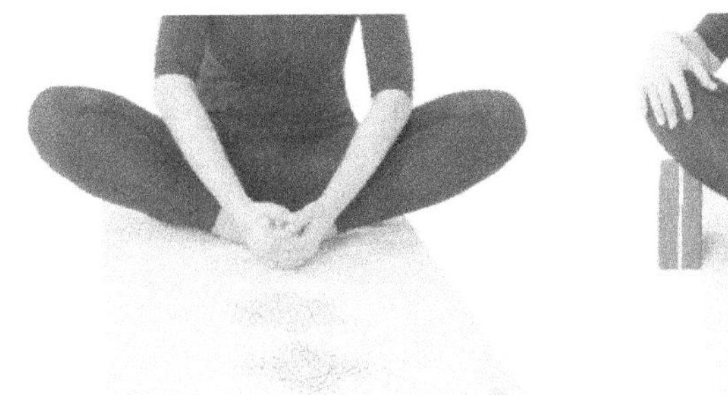 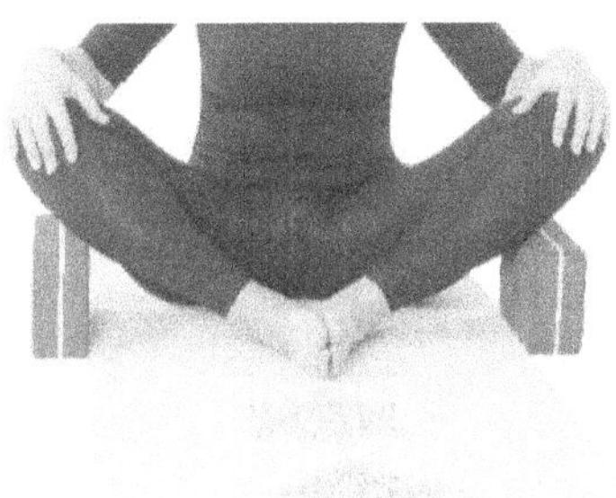

While in the base position, keep the head and spine straight, and the trunk stable. Use cushions or yoga blocks below the knees and hips for support if needed. Bend the knees, and bring the soles of the feet together, keeping the heels as close to the perineum as possible. If you are practising during pregnancy, keep them as far as possible from the perineum (approximately 1-foot distance or 30 centimetres or 12 inches). Position your hands either on top of the knees or grasp the knees, or grasp the toes, whichever feels more comfortable. Move the legs up and down in slow motion from the hips. The legs should move up to the maximum, or if you are pregnant, until the point the inner thighs are not hitting the belly. Try to bring the knees closer to the ground on the downward movement. Practise with a nice and smooth movement for 20-30 counts.

**Breathing:** Inhale while moving the legs upward and exhale when moving the legs downward.

**Benefits:** Can be practised both before and after meditative poses. It relieves tension from the muscles of the inner thighs and rests the legs.

**Precautions:** Those with sciatica and sacral conditions should avoid this exercise.

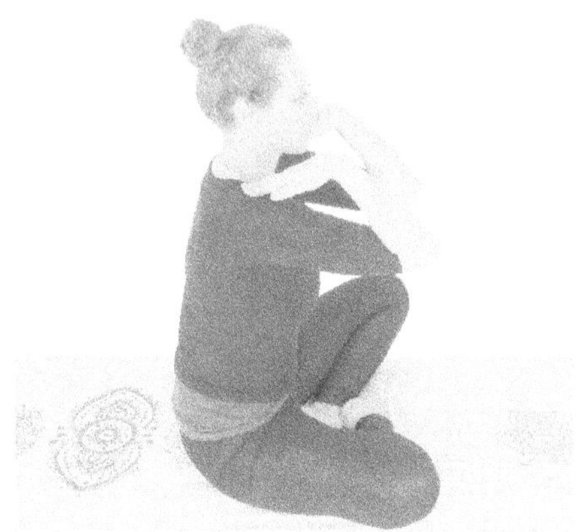

Bring your hands in front of your body with your palms facing the sky. Inhale and straighten the arms, exhale and bend the elbows to rest your fingers on your shoulders. Your upper arms should remain parallel to the ground and relaxed. Repeat for 5-10 counts with normal and continuous breathing/movement.

**Variation:**

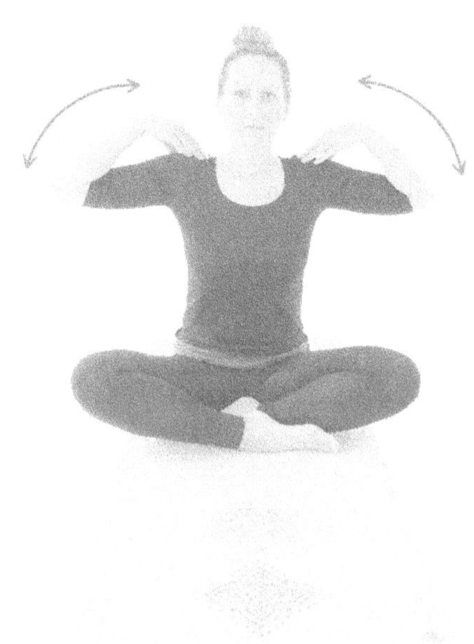

Extend your arms to the sides at shoulder level in a T-like shape with the hands open and palms facing the sky. Inhale and straighten the arms sideways, exhale and bend your elbows and rest your fingers on your shoulders. Your upper arms should remain parallel to the ground and relaxed. Repeat 5-10 times with continuous breathing/movement.

**Benefits:** Helps to correct body posture and stretches the ligaments to promote mobility and flexibility. It also strengthens the range of motion for those with chronic elbow conditions.

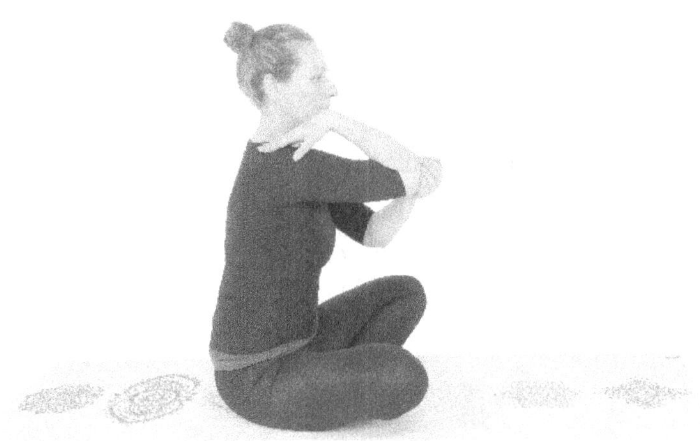

Touch the left shoulder with the fingers of the left hand and support the left arm by holding the elbow with the right hand. The left arm should be parallel to the ground in the starting position. Rotate the bent left elbow in a full circle so that both the lower arm and hand rotate together. The fingers of the left hand should be loose on the left shoulder so they move past the shoulder while rotating. Lower the left arm slowly and repeat the same with the right arm Move each arm clockwise and anticlockwise slowly and repeat 5-10 times.

**Breathing:** Inhale on the upward movement and exhale on the downward movement.

**Benefits:** Stimulates and at the same time relaxes the elbow joint.

# Exercise 51:   Shoulder socket rotation or Skandha Chakra

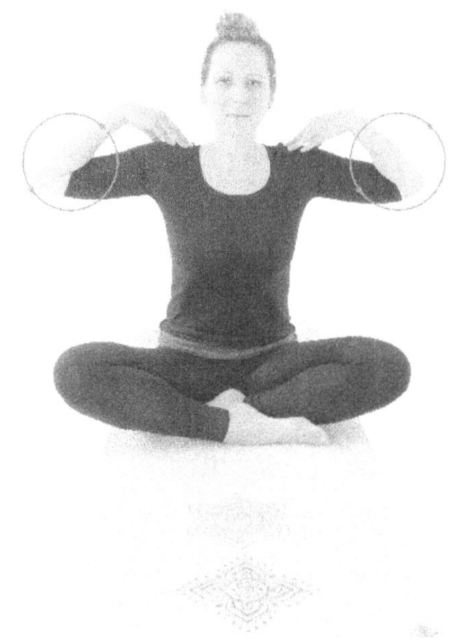

Touch the left shoulder with the fingers of the left hand and keep the right hand on the right knee with the spine erect. Rotate the left elbow in a full circle. On the forward movement, bring the elbow in front of the chest. On the upward movement, attempt to touch the left ear. On the backward movement, stretch the left arm back. On the downward movement, attempt to touch the left side of the trunk. Practice slowly 5-10 times, both clockwise and anticlockwise. Repeat the same on the right side.

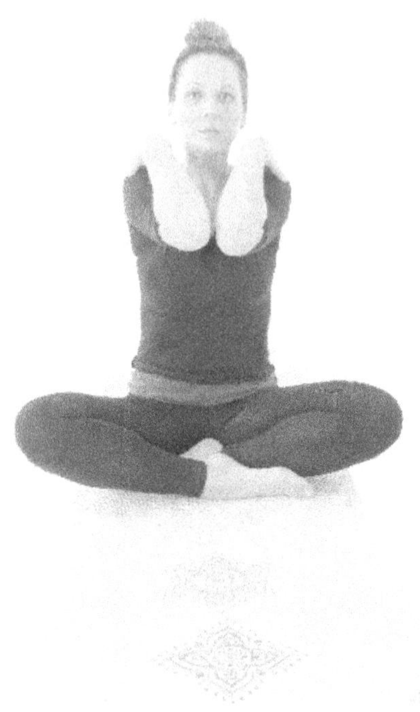

**Variation:** Touch the right shoulder with the fingers of the right hand and the left shoulder with the fingers of the left hand and rotate both elbows at the same time in a full circle. On the forward movement, attempt to touch the elbows in front of the chest. On the upward movement, attempt to touch the ears to allow the chest to open and stretch. On the backward movement, stretch the arms back. On the downward movement, attempt to touch the sides of the trunk. Practise slowly 5-10 times in both clockwise and anticlockwise directions.

**Breathing:** Inhale on the upward movement and exhale on the downward movement.

**Benefits:** Helps correct body posture and offers relief in cervical spondylitis and frozen shoulder. It also maintains the shape of the shoulders and chest and stimulates the respiratory system and oxygen flow in the body.

# Exercise 52:    Seated palm tree pose or Parvatasana in Sukhasana

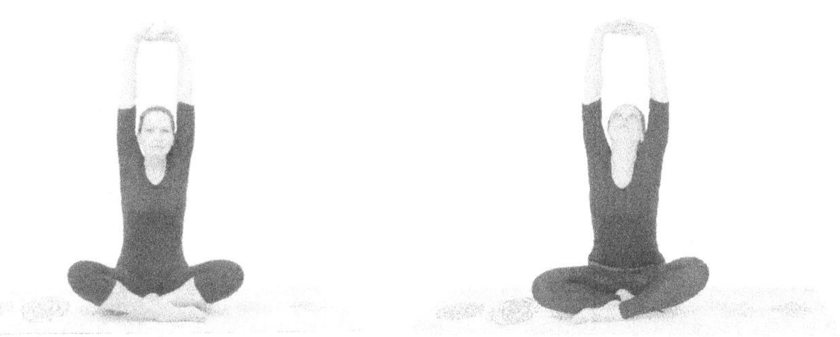

Sit up straight in a comfortable cross-legged position, interlock the fingers and inhale to lift your arms above the head with palms facing the sky. Fix your gaze either on your fingers above your head or straight ahead. This is the starting position. Stay in this position for 5-10 normal breaths. Repeat 2 times.

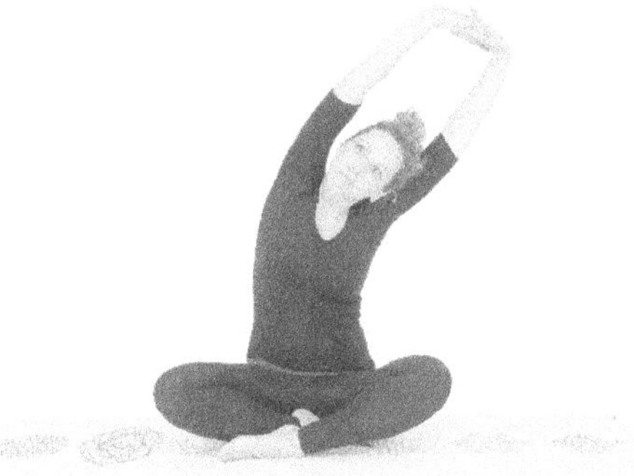

Exhale and bend sideways towards the left to feel the stretch on the right side of the rib cage. Inhale and return to the centre. Exhale and bend sideways to the right. Inhale and return to the centre. Repeat 5-10 times.

**Breathing:** Inhale and raise your hands, exhale while bending and inhale while coming back to the centre.

**Awareness:** Sacral (Swadhisthana) Chakra, Solar Plexus (Manipura) Chakra or Heart (Anahata) Chakra.

**Benefits:** This lateral bending is for the intercostal muscles. It strengthens the muscles in the arms, shoulders, chest, back, vertebrae, knees and psoas. Releases tension in the arms, shoulders, neck, spinal cord and rib cage. Gazing at the hands during practice can stimulate the eye muscles to reduce puffiness under the eyes and black circles. The pose also involves the upward movement of the head which helps balance the thyroid glands, tone the front of the neck and reduce the double chin.

**Precautions:** Those with sciatica, or severe conditions in the neck, shoulders, back or knees should avoid this practice. If you are suffering from nausea or dizziness do not gaze at the hands, instead look straight during the practice.

## Exercise 53:   Seated side bend or Parsva Sukhasana

Start with both hands at the knees. Position the left hand flat on the ground or take the support of a yoga block. The position of the hand should be on the side of the left buttock or lower limb, next to the knee.

Inhale to raise the right arm, bending the left elbow close to the rib cage. Exhale and bend sideways towards the left side. The hand can either be lengthened in a straight line or curved. Inhale and come back to the centre. Repeat 5-10 times on each side.

**Variation 1:** Inhale and take your hands up, exhale and bend the elbows. Hold your elbows with the opposite hands. Breathe normally and feel the stretch in the chest region. Fix your head between the upper arms. Exhale and bend sideways towards the left, inhale and come to the centre, exhale and bend sideways towards the right, and finally, inhale to come back to the centre. Repeat 5-10 times.

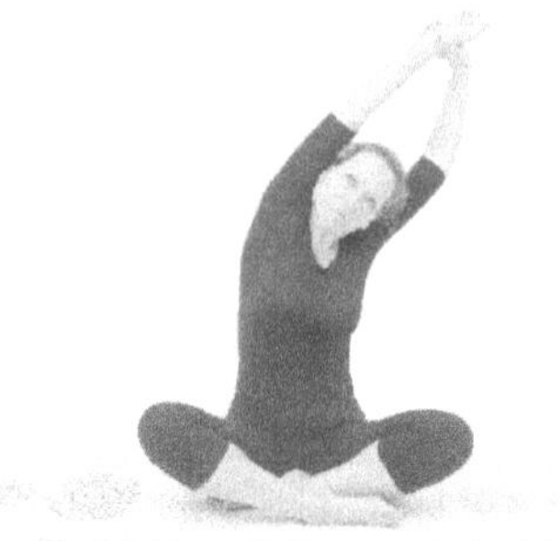

**Variation 2:** Inhale and raise both hands with palms facing forward. With the left hand grasp the wrist of the right hand to lengthen the arm. Exhale and bend sideways towards the left to feel the stretch on the side of the rib cage. Inhale and return to the centre. Change your hands, hold the left wrist with the right hand. Exhale and bend sideways to the right. Inhale and return to the centre. Repeat 5-10 times.

**Breathing:** Inhale and raise your hands, exhale and bend, and inhale and come back to the centre.

**Awareness:** Sacral (Swadhisthana) Chakra, Solar Plexus (Manipura) Chakra or Heart (Anahata) Chakra.

**Benefits:** This is lateral bending for the intercostal muscles. It can also benefit the muscles in the arms and shoulders, chest, back and vertebrae, knees, and psoas. It can release the tension in the neck and help balance the thyroid glands

**Precautions:** Those with sciatica, or severe conditions in the areas of neck, shoulders, back or knees should avoid this exercise.

# Exercise 54:   Seated spinal twist or Parivritti Sukhasana

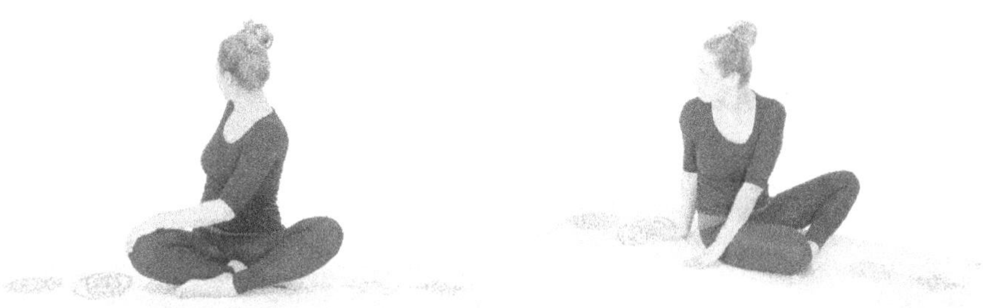

Sit up straight in a comfortable cross-legged position and breathe normally. Inhale and exhale to rest the right hand on the left knee. Inhale and place the left hand near your lower back or slightly away from the buttocks. Your head should be turned towards the left shoulder. Exhale and return to the centre. Repeat the same on the other side to complete 1 round. Repeat 5-10 times.

**Breathing:** Controlled breathing in line with the movement.

**Awareness:** Sacral (Swadhisthana) Chakra or Root (Mooladhara) Chakra.

**Benefits:** This open twist stretches the hips, knees, and ankles. It increases flexibility throughout the chest, shoulders and spinal cord and loosens the vertebrae. It releases the tension in the posterior muscles and helps remove stress, stimulates the diaphragm and digestive system and can relieve mild backache. It also tones the sides of the neck.

**Precautions:** Those with neck, shoulders, spine, lower back, hips, knees or pelvic floor conditions should only practice in the presence of an experienced yoga teacher.

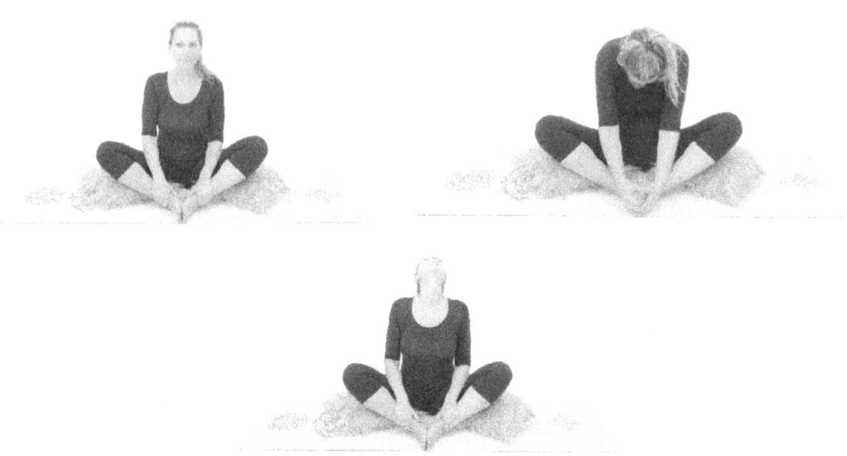

Sit comfortably with your spine erect either in a cross-legged position or in the full butterfly pose (Poorna Titali Asana). You can use cushions or yoga blocks for support under each thigh or knee if required. The hands can be either on the ankles or on the toes. Inhale, open the chest and look up with a mildly curved back. Exhale, drop the chin to the chest and round the back gently. Repeat 5-10 times.

**Breathing:** Synchronized breathing along with the movement. Inhale and open the chest and exhale while rounding the back.

**Awareness:** Heart (Anahata) Chakra or Throat (Vishuddhi) Chakra.

**Benefits:** Stretches the front of the neck, chest, shoulder and entire upper arm. The same benefits apply even in the cross-legged position. The stretch of the neck reduces the double chin, shapes the jawline and tones the chest.

**Precautions:** You should only practise while seated on a chair if you suffer from sciatica or pelvic conditions.

# Exercise 56:   Seated camel pose or Ushtrasana in Sukhasana

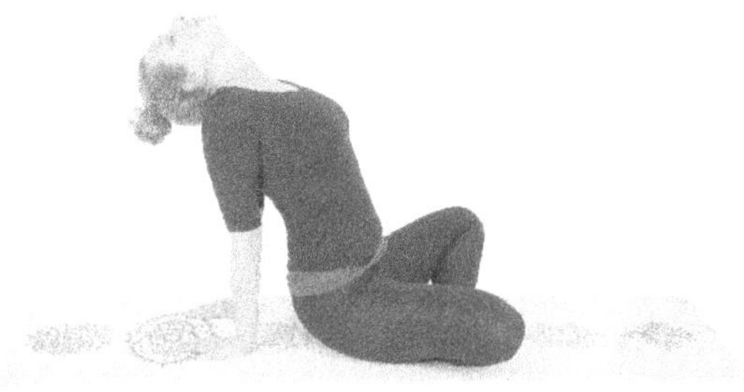

Sit in a comfortable cross-legged position and rest your hands on the ground behind the buttocks at a comfortable distance. Your spine should be in the neutral erect position. Inhale and move your hands slightly further away from the buttocks, then exhale. Inhale and expand the chest, and create a gentle backward bend while allowing your head to follow the movement by dropping back. Stay in that position while breathing normally for 10-15 easy counts. Inhale, exhale and bring the hands closer to the buttocks and gently bring the upper body back to the centre. Repeat 5-10 times.

**Breathing:** Normal breathing between the moves. Inhale and adjust the hands behind the buttocks, inhale and expand the chest and drop the head back. Exhale to come back to the centre.

**Awareness:** Heart (Anahata) Chakra or Throat (Vishuddhi) Chakra.

**Benefits:** Stretches the chest, shoulder blades, spinal cord and entire upper arm. The drop of the head tones the throat, neck area and double chin. Blood flows to the head to give you a glowing face.

**Precautions:** Not to be practised by those with conditions affecting the wrists.

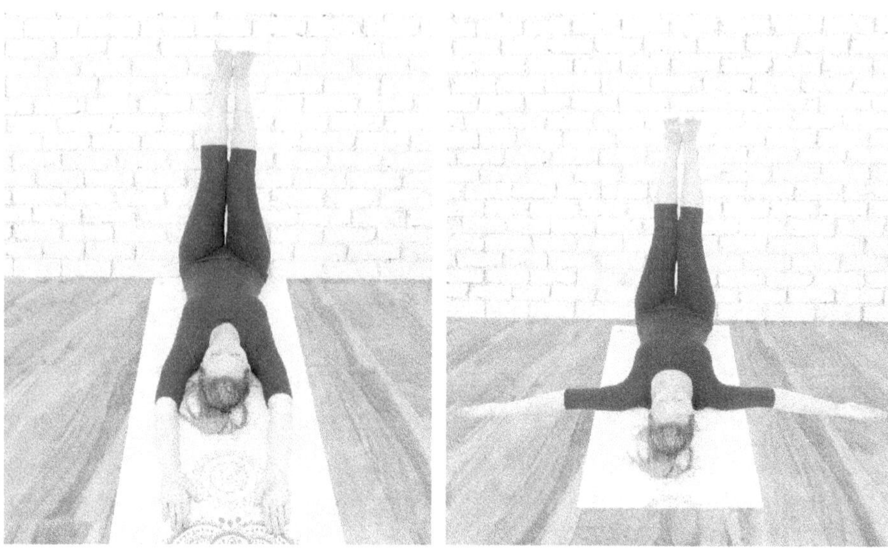

This is a gentle restorative asana. You can place props such as soft pillows or cushions and folded blankets close by to support the body if needed.

Position yourself near a wall with your legs outstretched and the left side of your body touching the wall. Inhale and as you exhale lie on your back and gently move your legs up against the wall with the soles of the feet facing upwards. The feet should be comfortably apart so that the muscles remain unengaged in holding them. The hands can be placed on the side of the trunk, extended behind the head or open in a T-shape, or in any other comfortable pose.

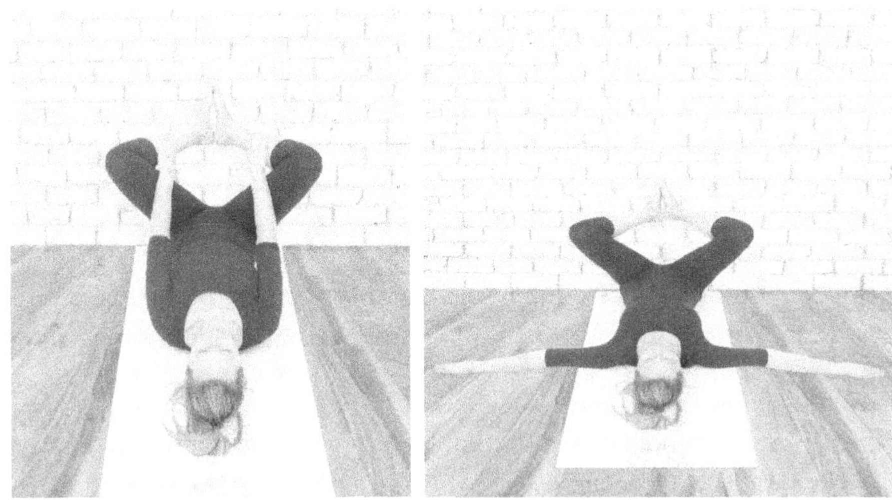

Alternatively, to increase the stretch, bend the knees and touch the soles of your feet. Then, slide the outer edges of the feet down and bring the heels closer to the pelvic floor. Adjust your body to a comfortable position, by moving the buttocks away from the wall if needed. Your back and head should continue to rest on the ground. The head and the neck should be in a neutral position, facing up to the sky, and the throat and the face must be calm and relaxed. Close your eyes and breath normally or practise a pranayama technique if you are familiar with them. You should hold the position for at least 5 minutes. When you are ready to release the pose, exhale and roll to any one side. Inhale to sit up.

**Breathing:** Normal breathing or practise Pranayama breathing techniques.

**Duration:** 5-20 minutes

**Benefits:** Soothes and calms the mind. Promotes the energy of prana movement and blood circulation from the legs to the upper centre of the body. It prevents varicose veins, oedema and swollen feet, and relaxes tired and cramped feet and the pelvic floor. It is a great stretch for the front of the torso, hamstrings, lower back and the back of the neck and strengthens capillary circulation in the facial muscles, making the facial skin look fresher and younger. It also promotes relaxation in the heart and increases your body's metabolism which results in fat reduction around the waist.

**Therapeutic benefits:** Relieves the nervous system and reduces stress, anxiety, and insomnia, helps with headaches, migraine, arthritis, and digestive disorders, and balances blood pressure. The longer the duration of the practice, the better the results for a rejuvenated body and mind.

**Precautions:** Should be avoided by women on lochia or during menstruation. Not to be practised by those with glaucoma or other severe eye conditions. Others with serious back and neck conditions should practice only in the presence of a certified yoga teacher and with the use of props as a support system.

**Note:** If during practice a tingling is experienced in the feet, bend the knees and touch the soles and bring the heels closer to the pelvic floor.

Healthy nutrition, frequent exercise and good sleep will increase the youthfulness and vitality of your body. When it comes to face yoga, as a rule, you can assume that if your digestive system is malfunctioning, it will show on your face commonly in the form of dryness, acne or pimples. The most effective yoga asanas that impact your face are the inverted poses and all those that regulate the digestive system as well as the nervous system. Blood circulation will regulate the function of all glands and organs, therefore our skin too. Any inverted asana will improve the flow of blood to the head and help your skin glow, and make it look and be healthier.

Moreover, exercise does not strengthen the muscles alone! Amongst others, exercise improves the functioning of the nerves that serve the muscles and other body parts. When you work out, the activity on the peripheral nervous system is what tones and strengthens the nerves, just like in the case of muscle strengthening.

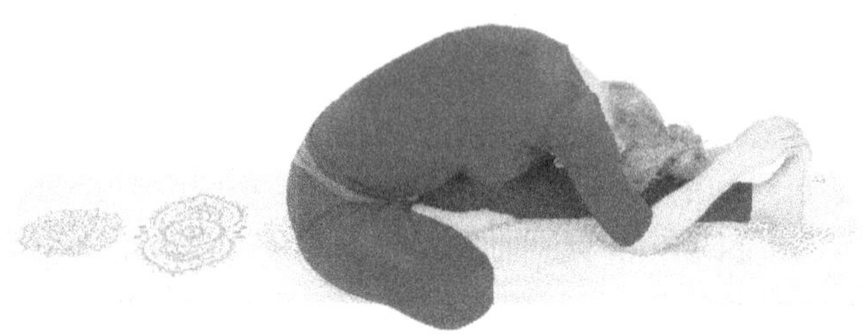

Sit with your legs stretched out in front of your body with your feet together. Bend the right leg, place the heel against your perineum or as close to it as possible and keep the knee grounded. Your left leg remains stretched out. Place your hands on the left knee with your spine erect and your back relaxed. This is the starting position. Slide your hands down the left leg to bend forward, try to reach for your toes and grasp them with both hands. Try to touch the knee with your forehead. This is the final position. Hold the position for as long as it feels comfortable with your back relaxed. Inhale and return to starting position. Repeat the same with the other leg. Repeat 3-5 times per side.

**Breathing:** Inhale at starting position, exhale and bend forward. Breathe normally if you are holding the position for long. Inhale and return to the starting position.

**Benefits:** Same as Paschimottanasana. It relaxes the muscles of the lower limbs.

**Details:** Same as Paschimottanasana. This is a preparatory asana for Paschimottanasana, meditation poses and the rest of the asanas.

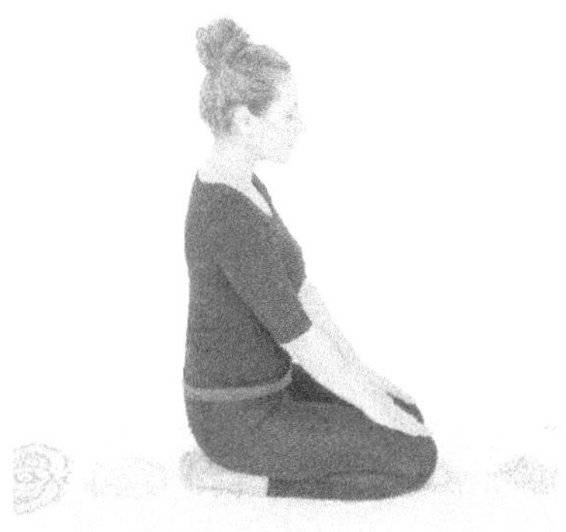

Kneel and sit between your heels while the big toes touch each other.

**Modification:**

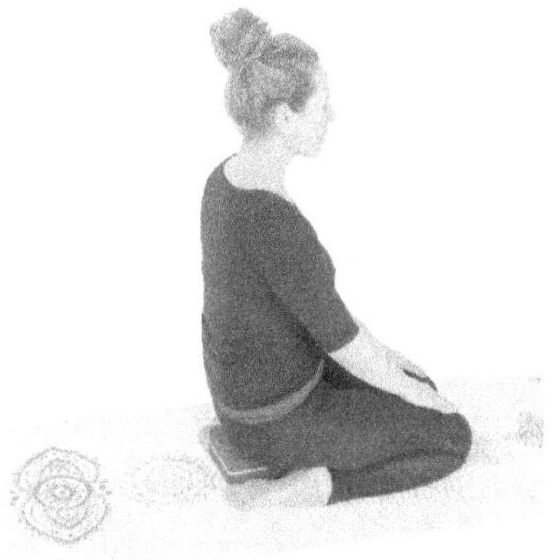

If you cannot sit comfortably in this position, place a yoga block or a folded towel under your buttocks. With this, your feet will need to be adjusted and open to accommodate the prop being used.

**Benefits:** Practice this pose after a meal for at least 5 minutes to directly stimulate your digestive function. A well-functioning digestive system is indirectly related to the health of your skin and hair and makes the skin glow.

**Awareness:** Solar Plexus (Manipura) Chakra.

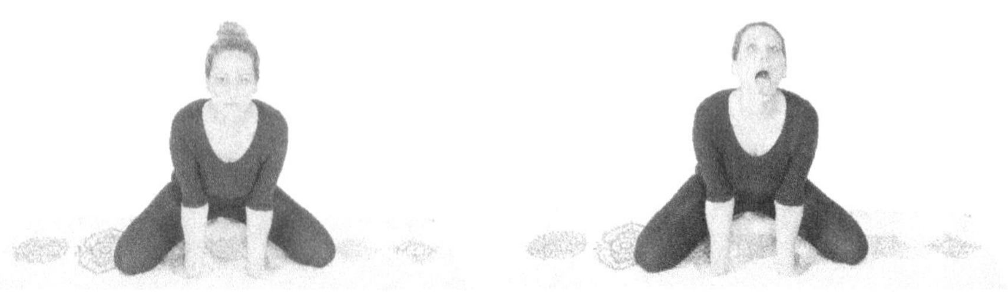

From Vajrasana, open your knees and maintain contact between the toes. Lean forward and place your palms in front of your body, with your fingers facing you. Stretch your body and keep your back arched. Gaze at the centre of your eyebrows with your eyes open. Inhale and bring your tongue out as far as possible, in an attempt to mimic a roaring lion. Slowly exhale through the mouth and make an 'aaa' sound from the throat while the tongue is still out and the mouth wide open. Your breath capacity is your limit, do not force the breath or the sound. Close the mouth at the end of inhalation and take 1-2 breaths before repeating the same. Repeat 5-10 times.

**Benefits:** The parts that benefit from this asana are the face, eyes, ears, nose, mouth, tongue, vocal cords, throat, chest, respiratory tract, diaphragm, abdomen, hands and fingers. It relaxes the facial muscles and helps reduce stress, anxiety, depression, anger, and tension on the face and its parts. It also helps with bleary or burning eyes, and delays ageing by removing wrinkles and stimulating the throat muscles to keep them firm as we age. It can cure stuttering, teeth grinding, and clenched jaws and helps get rid of bad breath. It exercises the tongue as it is fully stretched outside the mouth. It relaxes the neck muscles, relieves back pain and helps reduce stress and tension in the chest and diaphragm, getting rid of any respiratory tract infections. It enhances memory and poor concentration which makes it ideal for students, pregnant ladies and those who lack concentration. Those who use their voice as a profession can improve their voice tone and texture. It improves blood circulation, which in turn can restore energy to tired cells. When blood flow is more than sufficient across the body, you end up with glowing skin. In the traditional form of Hatha yoga, it is advisable to practice this pose in the healing rays of sunrise.

**Precautions:** None of the tongue exercises should be practised if you are suffering from face or tongue conditions. The roaring lion pose should not be practised during the first trimester and if you are suffering from knee or ankle-related conditions or osteoarthritis.

**Awareness:** Third-Eye (Ajna) Chakra or Throat (Vishuddhi) Chakra.

**Variation:** You can also practise the tongue side-to-side pose while in this position and produce the sound 'aaa.'

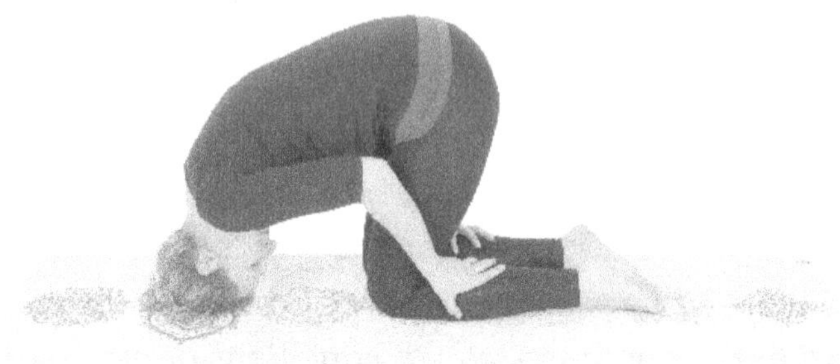

Sit in Vajrasana and grasp your calves just above your ankles. Slowly bend forward and place the crown of your head on the mat just in front of your knees. Raise the buttocks by keeping your thighs in an upright position and bring your chin closer to your chest. Stay in this position for 5-20 seconds. To return to Vajrasana, lower your buttocks, open your knees, place your palms between your thighs, raise your trunk and stay there for a few breaths. Repeat 5-10 times.

**Breathing:** Normal and soft breathing throughout the exercise.

**Awareness:** Crown (Sahasrara) Chakra.

**Benefits:** Rejuvenates the whole body and mind, relieves anxiety, reverses the blood flow to the head and face and helps with tissue regeneration, leading to a glowing face.

**Precautions:** Those with neck conditions, vertigo, high blood pressure or during pregnancy should not practice this exercise.

**Counter-pose:** Palm tree pose or Tadasana


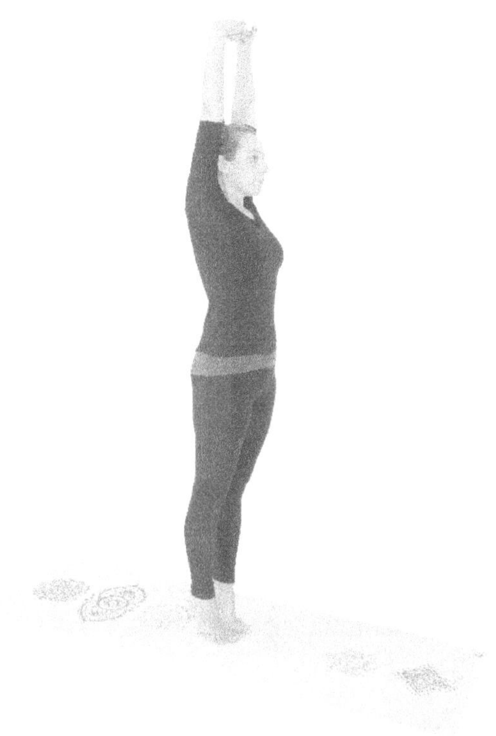

## Exercise 62:   Cat and cow stretch pose or Marjariasana

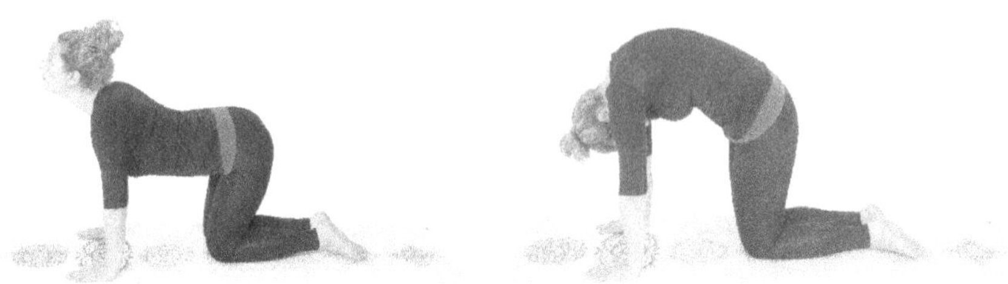

Sit in Vajrasana, then come on to all fours with the knees under the hips and your palms beneath your shoulders with your hands in front of the knees. This is the starting position.

Inhale while raising the head and curve your spine downwards. Expand the abdomen and fill your lungs with the maximum amount of oxygen. Hold your breath for 3 seconds. Exhale while lowering the head facing the thighs and arch the spine upwards, mimicking a cat's stretch. At the end of exhalation, engage your abdomen and the buttocks. This is 1 round. Repeat 5-10 times.

**Breathing:** Inhale and raise your head, exhale and lower your head.

**Awareness:** Sacral (Swadhisthana) Chakra.

**Benefits:** Improves the flexibility of the neck, shoulders and spine. Tones the neck muscles, double chin and jawline. It prepares the body for both forward and backward bends.

**Precautions:** If you are pregnant, you should not engage the abdomen. Those with neck, wrists, knees or ankles conditions should avoid this asana.

## Exercise 63:  Tiger pose or Vyaghrasana

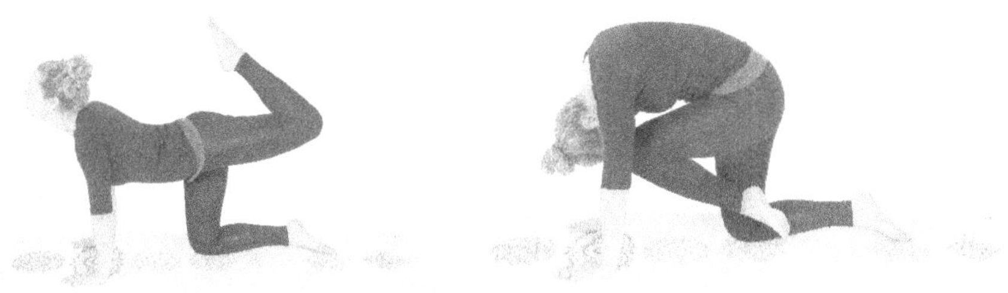

Get on all fours and look forward. Inhale while raising the head to curve the spine downwards, lift the left leg, bend it at the knee and try to touch the left heel to the left buttock or even higher towards the back of the head. Hold your breath in this position for 3-5 seconds.

Exhale while lowering the head and at the same time arch the spine upwards and give space for your leg to swing under the hips in an attempt to touch your knee to your nose. Hold your breath in this position for 3-5 seconds. This is 1 round. Repeat 10-20 times per side.

**Breathing:** Inhale and raise your head and leg and exhale to lower your head and leg.

**Awareness:** Sacral (Swadhisthana) Chakra.

**Benefits:** Improves the flexibility of the neck, shoulders, spine, back and hips. Tones the spinal nerves and abdominal muscles, double chin and jawline. It is a weight-reducing practice for the hips and thighs.

**Precautions:** If you are pregnant, swing the leg sideways from the hips to avoid any contact with the growing belly. Those with neck, wrist, knee or ankle conditions should avoid this asana.

# Exercise 64:   Child's pose or Shashankasana

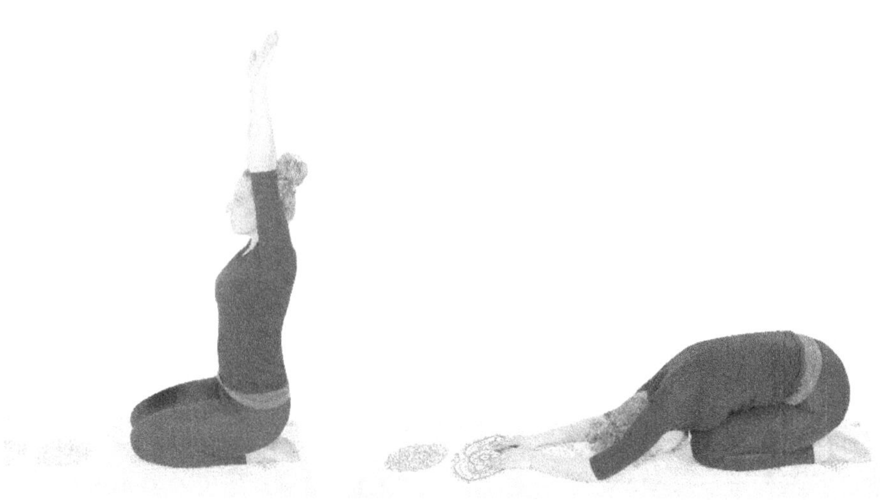

Sit in Vajrasana/Virasana, inhale and raise your hands. While exhaling, slowly bend the body forward from the hips so that the hands and the forehead can rest on the ground in front of the knees. You can use one or two cushions or a yoga block to rest the forehead if needed. Relax the forearms slightly and keep them flat on the ground. When in the final position, breathe normally and take 2 deep and long breaths. To release the pose, inhale and slowly, without any jerky movements, raise your arms and trunk to reach Vajrayana. Exhale and bring your hands to your knees. This is 1 round. You can practice 3-5 rounds.

**Breathing:** Inhale to raise your hands. Exhale to bend your body forward. Breathe normally.

**Duration:** Practice for 3-10 minutes and hold the final position comfortably.

**Awareness:** Solar Plexus (Manipura) Chakra or Sacral (Swadhisthana) Chakra

**Benefits:** Helps open the pelvic muscles and the sciatic nerves. Removes tension and pain from the lower back. Helps realign the spine. Creates space around the belly during pregnancy. It is a soothing and energizing asana which relieves nausea.

**Contraindications:** Those who suffer from vertigo or nausea, very high blood pressure and back conditions should avoid this asana.

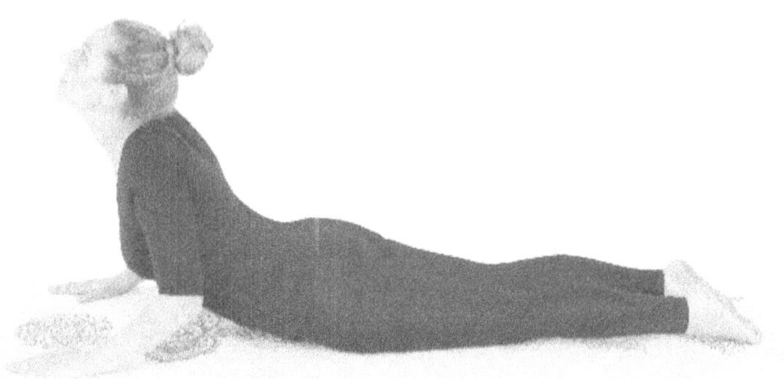

Lie flat on your stomach with your legs straight and feet together. Place your palms slightly to the side of your shoulders. Your arms should be close to the side of the body and the elbows slightly bent. Rest your forehead on the mat, close your eyes and relax your whole body, particularly the lower back. This is the starting position.

Raise your head slowly, compressing the muscles of the neck and the shoulders. Straighten the elbows and use your back and arm muscles to lift and open the chest and arch the back. Hold the final position for as long as it feels comfortable. To get out of the position, first lower the bent arms, navel, chest, shoulders and at last the forehead onto the mat. Be aware of your lower back and relax the muscles for a few breaths. Repeat 5-10 times.

**Breathing:** Inhale while raising the chest. Breathe normally or hold your breath while in position. Exhale while lowering the chest.

**Awareness:** Sacral (Swadhisthana) Chakra.

**Benefits:** Improves breathing and helps with spinal flexibility, backache, as well as gynaecological disorders. It also stimulates the appetite, alleviates constipation and tones the hips and thighs. When your chin points forward, the neck muscles get toned, and the double chin and the jawline are shaped.

**Precautions:** Avoid practising if you suffer from hyperthyroidism, hernia, peptic or intestinal disorders.

**Note:** The pubic bone should be on the floor and the navel raised to ~3 cm maximum, otherwise the knees will be strained. Straighten your arms as per the flexibility of your back. The aim is not to straighten the arms but to open the chest.

## Exercise 66:   Bow pose or Dhanurasana

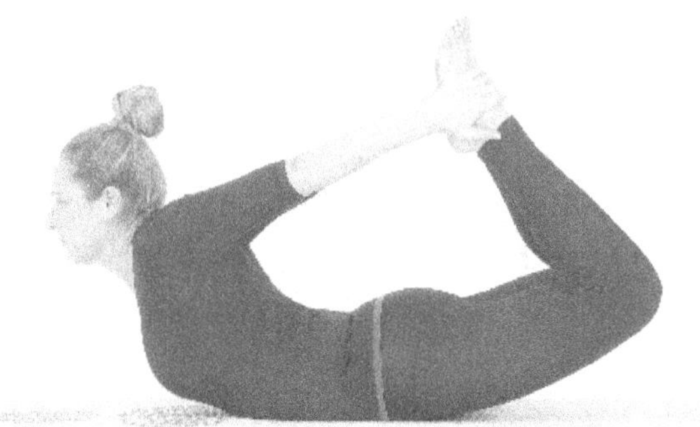

Lie flat on your stomach. Keep your feet together and your hands beside your body. Bend the knees as close to the buttocks as possible and grasp the ankles with your hands. Your chin should be on the floor. This is the starting position.

Inhale and hold your breath to push the feet away from the body and arch your back by lifting the thighs, chest and head together with the arms straight. In the final position, your head is tilted back and your whole body is supported by the abdomen. Your upper leg muscles should be engaged to help you balance on your abdomen. Your back and arms should be relaxed. Remain in this position for as long as it feels comfortable or breathe slowly by rocking the body gently to follow the breath. Exhale and come out of the position by slowly lowering your legs, chest and head to the starting position. Release the pose and relax in a prone position until your breath returns to normal. Repeat 5-10 times.

**Breathing:** Inhale in starting position. Hold your breath while raising the body. Breathe slowly and deeply in synchronization with a slow and gentle rocking movement on the body in the final position. If this is challenging, hold your breath. Exhale to come out of the position.

**Awareness:** Solar Plexus (Manipura) Chakra or Third-Eye (Ajna) Chakra.

**Benefits:** This is an asana which can be done in the morning as it stimulates the adrenal glands which produce hormones that you need to regulate the metabolism, immune system, and blood pressure. Their secretion is better balanced when you are awake and the sympathetic nervous system increases the heart rate and gives you energy for the day ahead. It also stretches, removes stiffness and tones the whole body, particularly the thighs and improves breathing. As the chin points forward, the neck muscles get toned, while also shaping the double chin and the jawline. The kidneys, liver and digestive system are also massaged, improving their general functioning. It also improves blood circulation and oxygen flow in the whole body and amongst all its benefits, helps your face glow.

**Precautions:** Avoid practising if you suffer from high blood pressure or heart conditions, hernia, colitis, or digestive disorders.

# Exercise 67:  Camel pose or Ushtrasana

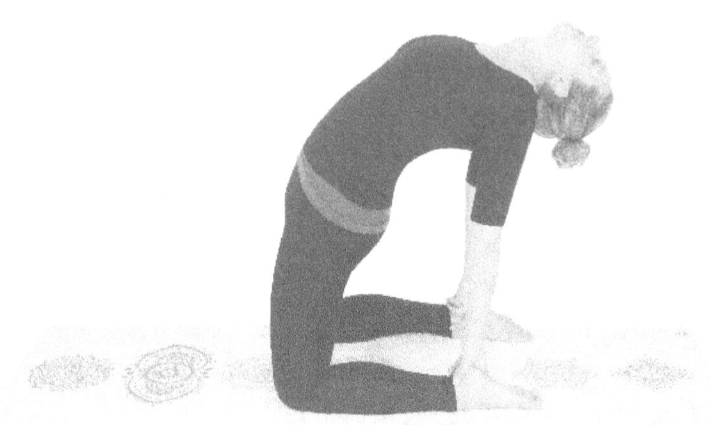

Stand on your knees which are placed hip-width apart while breathing normally until the position feels comfortable. Keep your knees and feet apart to maintain balance. The toes should be flat on the ground. Sit upright with the trunk straight and breathe normally. Bring both hands behind the hips or at the lower back level if that feels comfortable. Find your balance and position of comfort while breathing normally. This is the starting position.

Inhale to gently push the hips forward. As the upper body leans backwards, touch the left heel with the left hand and the right heel with the right hand. The hips should be pushed forward slightly and the head and spine slightly backward until the comfort zone is reached. Stay in this position for as long as you feel comfortable and breathe normally. To come back to the centre, slowly release one hand at a time from the heels, bring the head up and lean forward to bring the body to an upright position. Repeat up to 3 times.

**Breathing:** Normal and soft breathing throughout the exercise.

**Awareness:** Sacral (Swadhisthana) Chakra or Throat (Vishuddhi) Chakra.

**Benefits:** This asana is beneficial for the reproductive system during the preconception period. It stimulates the digestive system and stretches the stomach, and intestines while preventing constipation. The vertebrae get relaxed with the backward bend and the spinal nerves get stimulated. It can relieve backache and postural problems like a rounded back and dropping shoulders. The thyroid gland gets regulated as the throat and its organs are fully stretched which can also tone the double chin and jawline. Since this asana is a chest opener, it can benefit the respiratory system and expand the lungs. It is useful for those suffering from asthma and breathlessness, especially during pregnancy. It stretches the abdominal and pelvic regions too.

**Precautions:** Those with back or spinal conditions should practice this asana only in the presence of a qualified yoga teacher.

**Note:** Make sure the body is not over-bending and the back is not curved, especially if you are practising during your third trimester. The bending should not be forceful, bend as little or as much as your body allows so that you can breathe comfortably without any jerky movements or strain. This modification intends to open up the chest and not go all the way down.

**Counter-pose:** Child's pose or Shashankasana

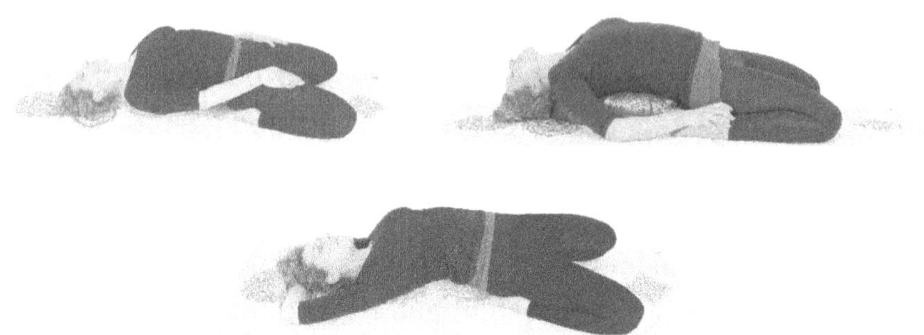

From Vajrasana, inhale and slowly bend back with the support of your elbows, one at a time. Exhale and bring the crown of the head to the ground while rounding up the back. If needed, separate the knees. When you balance on the position, keep your hands on the thighs or the ankles or the side of the body, or even under the back of the head with lesser benefit. The knees should remain in contact with the ground at all times if possible. Close your eyes and remain in the final position with slow and deep breathing for as long as it feels comfortable. There should be no strain during the practice. To release the pose, return to Vajrasana and then straighten your legs to avoid your knee joints from getting dislocated. Stay for a few seconds at the final position initially and then gradually increase the time.

**Breathing:** Slow breathing in the final position.

**Awareness:** Sacral (Swadhisthana) Chakra.

**Benefits:** Improves digestive and respiratory systems, strengthens and stretches the spinal muscles and nerves, and stretches and massages the quadriceps, ankles and the organs in the abdominal area. Offers pain relief for sciatica and also helps those suffering from high blood pressure. It relaxes and flexes the tendons and ligaments of the lower limbs and muscles of the knees. It stretches the chest increasing oxygen flow into the respiratory system which leads to a more relaxed face and healthier skin.

**Precautions:** Those with ankle, knee, hip, back, spinal, and neck conditions should avoid this asana or do it in the presence of an experienced yoga teacher. Use the support of a bolster to increase the inclination of the upper body. This asana should not be practised if you are suffering from abdominal hernia or other intestinal issues.

**Note:** If you are pregnant, you should practice only with the support of a bolster or cushions positioned across the spine as the inferior vena cava can be compressed, and the belly can be overstretched. You should not attempt to bring the crown of the head to the ground or arch the spine during pregnancy.

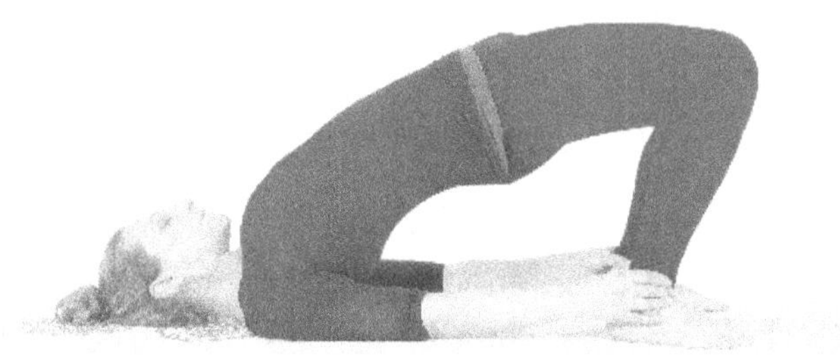

Lie in a supine position, bend your knees with the soles flat on the ground and your heels touching the buttocks or as close as possible. The feet and knees should be hip distance apart. Grasp your ankles with your hands. Adjust your shoulders to accommodate the position. This is the starting position.

Inhale and hold your breath to raise your buttocks and arch your back upwards. Raise the chest and navel like someone is pulling you up from the navel. Push the chest and try to touch the chin, without moving your feet or shoulders. Hold the position by holding your breath to your maximum extent. Exhale and lower the body by first releasing the ankles and then stretching your legs out. Repeat 5-10 times or as needed.

**Alternative:** Instead of holding the position, you can practice moving up and down in a continuous motion. Repeat 10-20 times.

**Breathing:** Inhale at the starting position. Hold your breath to raise your buttocks. Hold your breath in the final position or breathe slowly. Exhale to lower the body.

**Awareness:** Throat (Vishuddhi) Chakra or Heart (Anahata) Chakra.

**Benefits:** It can realign the spine and correct rounded shoulders. It also relieves backache and tones the abdomen, hip and thighs.

It improves digestion which indirectly affects the acne and pimples on the face and provides a glow.

**Precautions:** Not to be practised if you are suffering from an abdominal hernia and peptic or duodenal ulcers. During pregnancy and after the second trimester, do not raise the buttocks more than 15 cm and do not hold your breath.

# Exercise 70:    Fish pose or Matsyasana

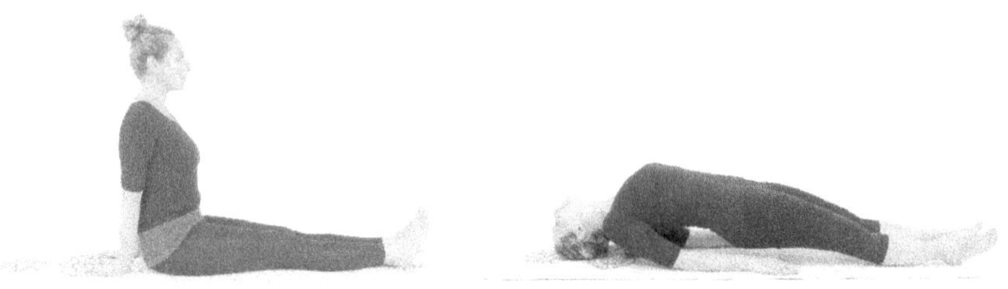

Sit at the base position or Prarambhik Sthiti and with the support of your hands and elbows lean backwards to rest your crown on the ground. Arch your back and place both your palms on the sides of your thighs with the lower arms resting on the ground. You can choose to lift your buttocks or sit on them. Stay in the final position for as long as it feels comfortable having engaged your hips, thighs, buttocks and abdomen. To return to starting position, lower your buttocks first, flatten your arms, shoulder and back of your neck and return your head to normal while in the supine position. Repeat up to 3 times.

**Breathing:** Slow and deep breathing in the final position.

**Awareness:** Solar Plexus (Manipura) Chakra or Heart (Anahata) Chakra.

**Benefits:** Stretches the intestines and abdominal organs, helps with inflamed and bleeding piles and supports the respiratory system through deep breathing. It also circulates blood to the whole body, particularly to the back and relieves backache. It also regulates the thyroid gland and stimulates the thymus gland which makes white blood cells that help boost the immune system and provide youthfulness, energy and strength.

**Precautions:** Not to be practised if you are suffering from high blood pressure, hernia, heart, peptic or back conditions.

**Note:** If you are suffering from constipation, it is recommended that you drink 3 glasses of water before practising this asana to soften bowel movement.

**Counter-pose:** Shoulder stand pose or Sarvangasana or plough pose or Halasana.

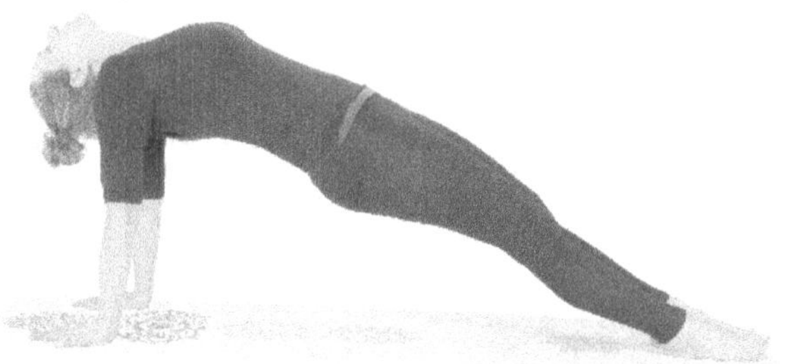

Sit with your legs stretched out in front of your body. Place your palms behind your buttocks about 30 cm away. Keep your elbows straight with the fingers pointing away from the back and the trunk slightly reclined. Inhale and raise the buttocks and lift the body. Exhale to let the head hang comfortably. Try to keep your soles flat on the ground. Keep your arms and legs straight and hold the position with normal breathing for a minimum of 45 seconds. [As you become stronger in that position, gradually increase the time]. To come out of the pose, exhale and lower your buttocks and sit. Rotate and stretch your wrists to relax them.

**Breathing:** Inhale to lift your body and exhale to hang your head. Continue with normal breathing while holding the position. Exhale to lower your body to starting position.

**Awareness:** Solar Plexus (Manipura) Chakra.

**Benefits:** Strengthens the shoulders, abdomen, thighs and wrists, and tones the back and spine, as well as the Achilles' tendons. The hanging of the head stretches the chest and neck to make the skin in these areas firm. Blood circulates to the head and gives you a glowing face. It also regulates the thyroid gland and stimulates the thymus gland which makes white blood cells that help boost the immune system and provide youthfulness, energy and strength.

**Precautions:** Not to be practised if you are suffering from high blood pressure, heart or stomach conditions, spondylitis, hernia or weak arms and wrists.

This practice is performed while in the hero's meditation pose or Dhyana Veerasana with the legs crossing over one another. If this seated position is not to your comfort, separate the legs and modify the practice and sit in Vajrasana.

Start by keeping the palms of your hands on your knees. Inhale and raise one hand and bend it over the opposite shoulder. Stretch the other hand to the side and bend it behind the back. The back of the hand should touch the spine while the opposite palm rests on the spine. Attempt to touch the fingers of both hands at the back. The raised elbow should be positioned behind the ear so that the head is resting on the inside of the raised arm. The head should be slightly back and the spine erect. Maintain the position for 3-5 comfortable breaths. Inhale and release the hand. Repeat the same with the other hand to complete 1 round. Repeat 5-10 times.

**Modification 1:**

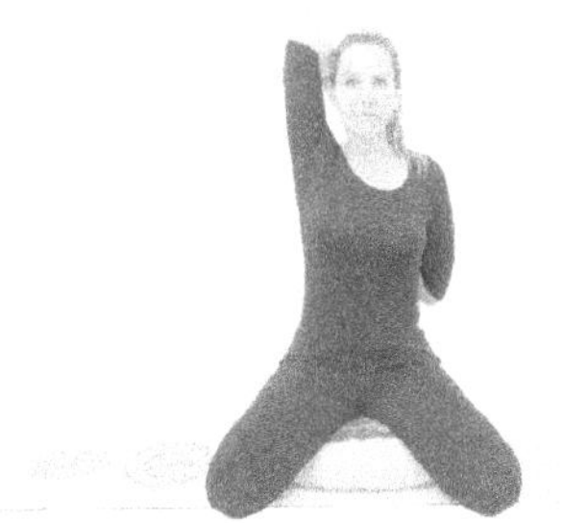

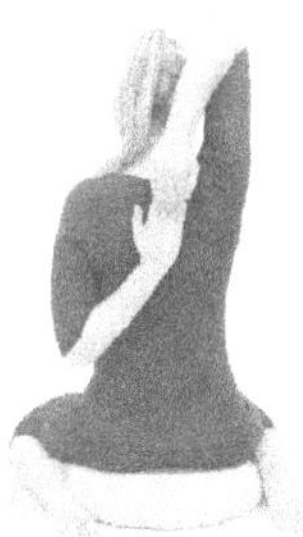

If you need to elevate the perineum, sit on a cushion to be comfortable in the position.

**Modification 2:**

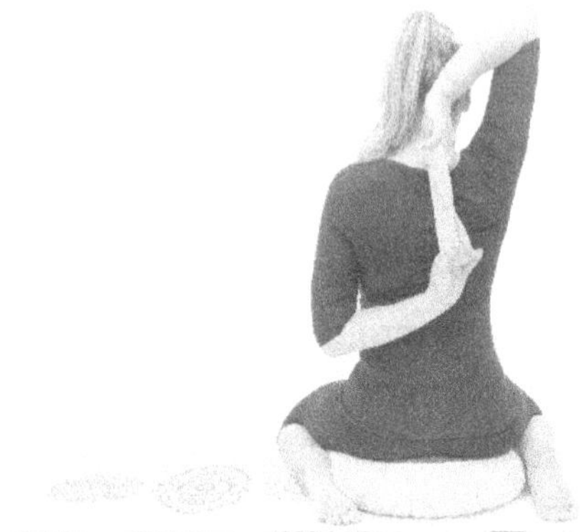

If you cannot touch the fingers of both hands, use a thera band or a cloth to hold the final position. This modified asana aims to open up the chest. Maintain the position of the head for a maximum stretch on the spine.

**Breathing:** Normal breathing.

**Awareness:** Third-Eye (Ajna) Chakra or Heart (Anahata) Chakra.

**Benefits:** This is a chest opening pose that stimulates the respiratory system, offers relief from backache, neck and shoulders stiffness, fatigue, tension, and anxiety and improves body posture. It also tones the neck and chest.

**Precautions:** Same as Vajrasana.

Sit in the staff pose or Dandasana. Relax your whole body. Inhale and as you exhale slowly bend forward from the hips, and slide your hands down toward your feet. Try to touch your toes or the soles of your feet, or any part of your legs that you can reach comfortably and without strain or breathing issues. Hold the position for a few seconds, then relax the back and legs to feel the stretch. To go deeper into the bend, maintain the position and use your arm muscles to bring the trunk toward your thighs. Try to touch your knees with your forehead. Hold this final position for as long as you can with deep and slow breathing. To release the pose, inhale to lift your body from the hips. Repeat 5-10 times.

**Modification:**

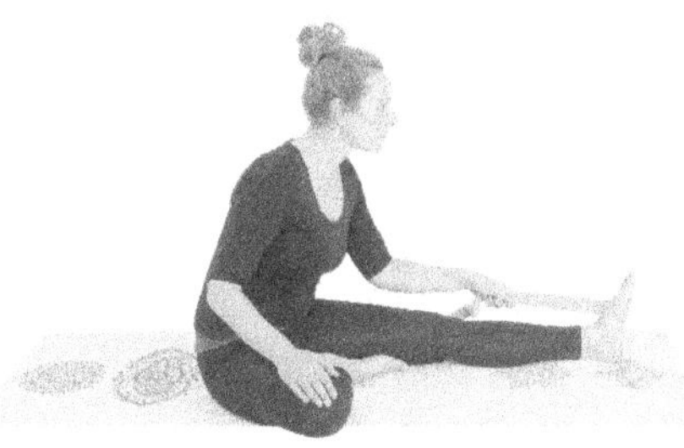

Take the support of a thera band if you need help to bend forward and reach deeper.

**Breathing:** Inhale at the starting position and exhale to bend. Inhale when you reach the position and exhale to go deeper on the forward bend. Breathe slowly and deeply at the final position. Inhale to release the pose.

**Awareness:** Sacral (Swadhisthana) Chakra.

**Benefits:** Increases flexibility in the hip joints and stretches the hamstrings. It also tones and massages the abdomen and pelvic region, as well as the internal organs in these areas. It stimulates blood circulation to the spine, head and face.

**Precautions:** Do not practice if you are suffering from a slipped disk, sciatica or hernia.

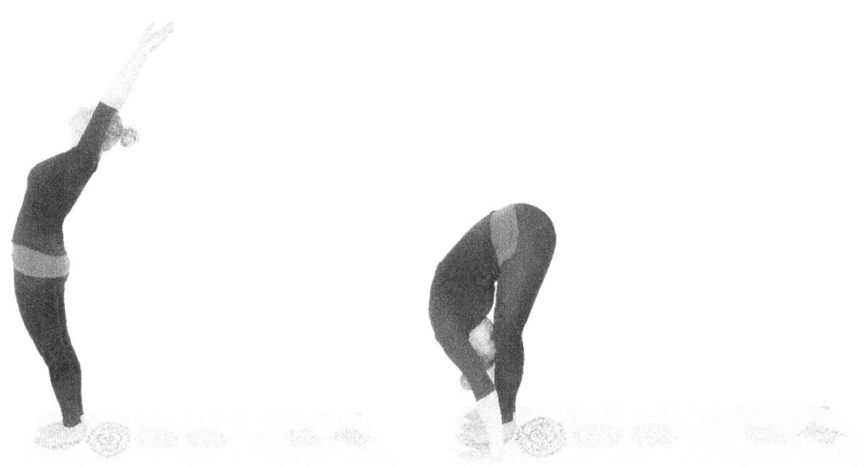

Begin with the raised arms pose or Hasta Utthanasana. Exhale and bend forward from the hips and touch the ground by the side of each foot with your fingers or palms. The forehead should come as close to the knees as it feels comfortable and the knees should be straight. Hold the position for 3-5 normal breaths. Inhale and straighten to come up to Hasta Utthanasana. Repeat 5-10 times.

**Modification:**

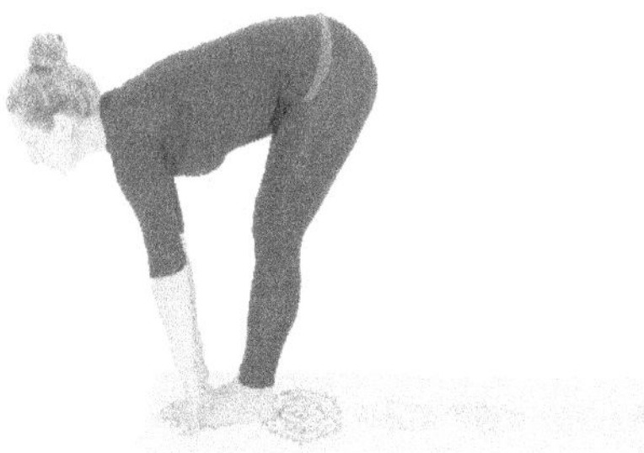

Those with back conditions should only bend from the hips to a maximum of 90 degrees or bend only to the point they feel comfortable. The spine should be straight. You can use the support of a yoga block or any other prop to take support for the hands.

**Breathing:** Exhale and bend forward. Contract the abdomen when in the final position and exhale as much air as possible from the lungs.

**Awareness:** Sacral (Swadhisthana) Chakra.

**Benefits:** Strengthens the spinal nerves. It can improve concentration and metabolism and blood circulation to the head and face. It massages the digestive organs and relieves you from flatulence, constipation, or indigestion. A balanced digestive system results in a glowing face.

**Precautions:** Do not practice if you are suffering from back conditions or high blood pressure.

# Exercise 75:   Mountain pose or Downward dog or Parvatasana

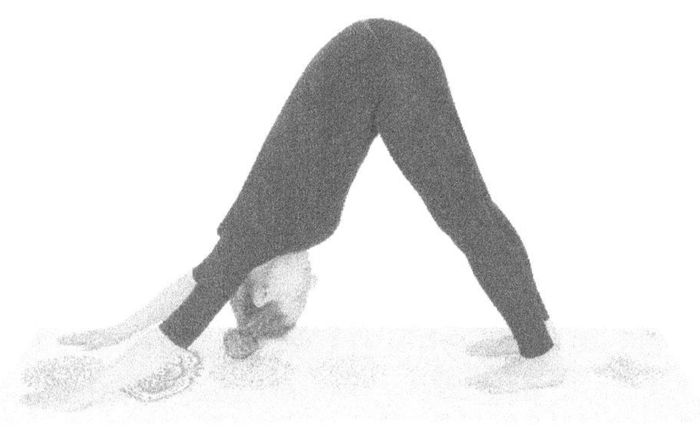

From a standing position, hold your body in a pyramid-like shape. Keep your hands still when in position, and slowly walk your feet back till both your soles are flat on the ground. Maintain the position with the legs and hands straight. Your head can either be between your upper arms or for maximum arm and spinal stretch, it can hang further inside your body reaching for the ground. The neck should be relaxed and straight while following the spinal motion. Stay in the position for as long as needed. To release the pose, bend the knees and come to Vajrasana. Repeat up to 3 times.

**Breathing:** Normal and soft breathing throughout the exercise.

**Awareness:** Throat (Vishuddhi) Chakra.

**Benefits:** Strengthens the muscles and nerves in your arms and legs. At a younger age, it helps increase your height as it stretches the muscles and ligaments so that bones can grow longer. It also enhances blood circulation in the area between the shoulder blades, head and face.

**Precautions:** Those with diseases of the brain, high blood pressure, blood conditions, heart conditions, back conditions, cervical or neck conditions, arteriosclerosis, glaucoma, and active ear infection as well as during menstruation or pregnancy, should not practice this asana.

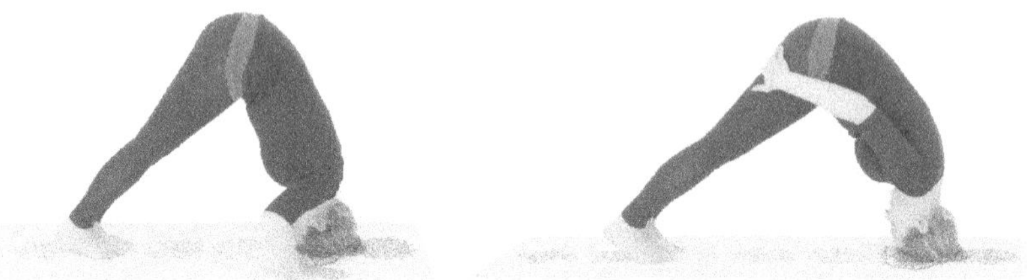

Begin by coming on all fours. Turn your toes to push your body weight forward. Bring your head to the ground and place your crown on the ground between your hands. Straighten your knees and raise your buttocks to balance on your crown and toes alone. Bring your feet together. Find your balance with the support of your hands, and slowly raise your arms to hold the sides of your buttocks. When you are balanced properly, come up higher on the toes. Hold the position for as long as this is comfortable. To release the pose, lower your arms beside your head and slowly return to all fours and then to the child's pose or Shashankasana to relax. This is 1 round. Practice up to the 3 rounds where you gradually increase the holding time of the pose.

**Modification:**

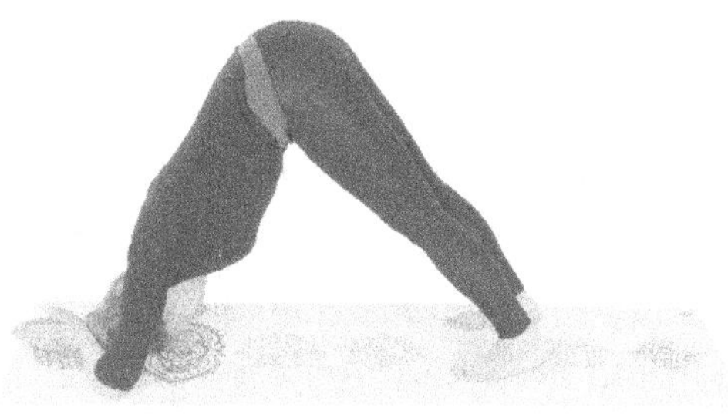

If you are unable to balance with your arms beside your buttocks, bring your palms to the Namaste Mudra in front of your head and hold that position for as long as possible.

**Breathing:** Normal and soft breathing throughout the exercise.

**Awareness:** Crown (Sahasrara) Chakra.

**Benefits:** Supplies more blood to the brain and activates the neurons. Helps with low blood pressure, balances the nervous system and strengthens the neck muscles.

**Precautions:** Those who have a cold or are suffering from vertigo, diseases of the brain, high blood pressure, blood conditions, heart conditions, back conditions, cervical or neck conditions, arteriosclerosis, glaucoma, active ear infection, weak eye capillaries, asthma, and during menstruation or pregnancy should not practice this asana.

**Counterpose:** After releasing the pose come to the child's pose or Shashankasana between your rounds of practice. Slowly come to the corpse pose or Shavasana for a couple of minutes and raise yourself to the palm tree pose or Tadasana.

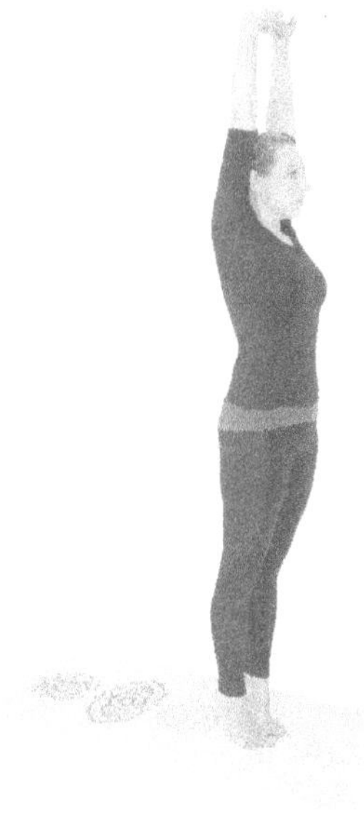

**Note:** Practice either the half headstand pose or Bhumi Pada Mastakasana or the crown based pose or Moordhasana.

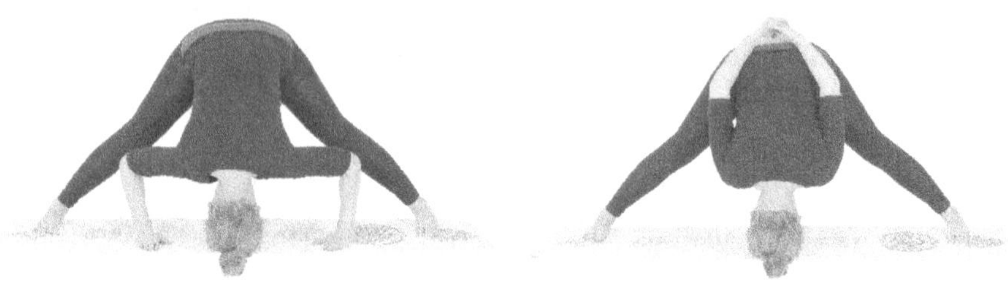

Begin from the mountain pose or downward dog or Parvatasana and bring your head towards the ground. Place your crown on the ground between your hands. To maintain your balance, adjust the legs and keep them far apart while your hands are still on the ground. Slowly raise your arms and bring them to your back by either holding onto one wrist with the other hand or interlocking your fingers. When you are balanced in the position, you can raise your heels and support your weight on your crown and toes only. Hold the position for as long as this is comfortable. To release the pose, lower your arms and keep them beside your head. Slowly return to Parvatasana, then to all your fours and then to child's pose or Shashankasana. This is 1 round. Practice up to the 3 rounds where you gradually increase the holding time of the pose.

**Breathing:** Normal and soft breathing throughout the exercise.

**Details:** Same as half headstand or Bhumi Pada Mastakasana.

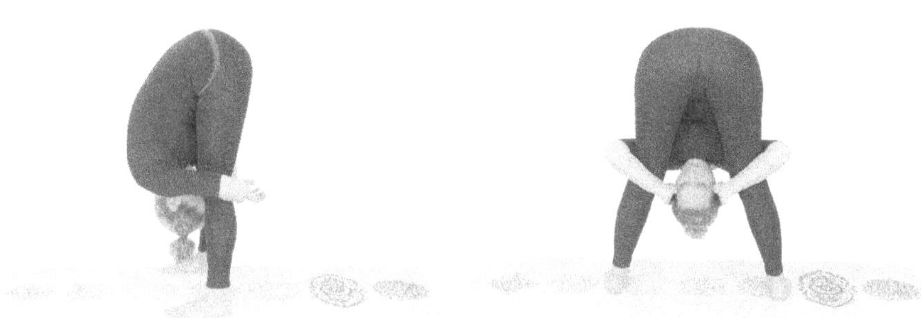

From a standing position, place your feet shoulder-width apart and place your arms beside your body. This is the starting position.

Stretch your arms in front of your chest and bend forward from the hips. Take your arms around your legs and either grasp them one wrist at a time or hook your hands behind the calves. Your head has to follow the forward bend. With the help of your arm muscles, bring the head closer or between your knees. Keep your legs straight. Rest your trunk against your thighs. Hold the final position for as long as it feels comfortable. To release the pose, first release the hands from behind your legs, then slowly raise your upper body and feel the movement of each vertebra. Stretch your arms in front of the chest before lowering them to starting position. Repeat 3-5 times.

**Breathing:** Inhale to stretch your arms in front of the chest. Exhale and retain breathing to bend forward and hold the final position. Inhale and return to the standing position with arms stretched out in front of the chest. Exhale to lower the arms.

**Awareness:** Sacral Chakra (Swadhisthana).

**Benefits:** Stimulates pancreatic function to result in sufficient insulin production, relaxes the hip joints, stretches the hamstrings, and massages the spinal nerves. It also rejuvenates the brain and revives the facial skin, cells and tissue.

**Precautions:** Do not practice this asana if you suffer from diseases of the brain, blood pressure, blood conditions, heart conditions, back conditions, cervical or neck conditions, arteriosclerosis, glaucoma, active ear infection as well as during menstruation or pregnancy.

**Counterpose:** Snake pose or Sarpasana, bridge pose or Setu Asana or bow pose or Dhanurasana.

Lie down on your stomach. Keep your legs straight and feet together. Bring your hands to your back and interlock your fingers on top of your buttocks. Place your chin on the ground. This is the starting position. Engage your lower back muscles to lift the upper body and raise the chest as far as possible from the ground. Push your hand further to the back and raise your arms as high as possible with no strain. Pretend that someone is pulling your arms from behind. Squeeze your shoulder blades to raise your chest higher if possible. Look ahead and hold the position for as long as it feels comfortable. Slowly return to the starting position. Release your hands and keep your arms by your sides and relax your whole body. Turn your head to one side with one of the cheeks on the ground. This is 1 round. Repeat 3-5 times.

**Breathing:** Inhale deeply in the starting position. Retain your breath to raise and hold the final position. Exhale and lower your upper body.

**Awareness:** Heart Chakra (Anahata).

**Benefits:** Same as cobra pose or Bhujangasana. Also, this is an alignment pose for the spine and rounded shoulders. It also strengthens the back muscles. When engaging the front of your neck during this practice, you help with the reduction of a double chin.

**Precautions:** Same as cobra pose or Bhujangasana.

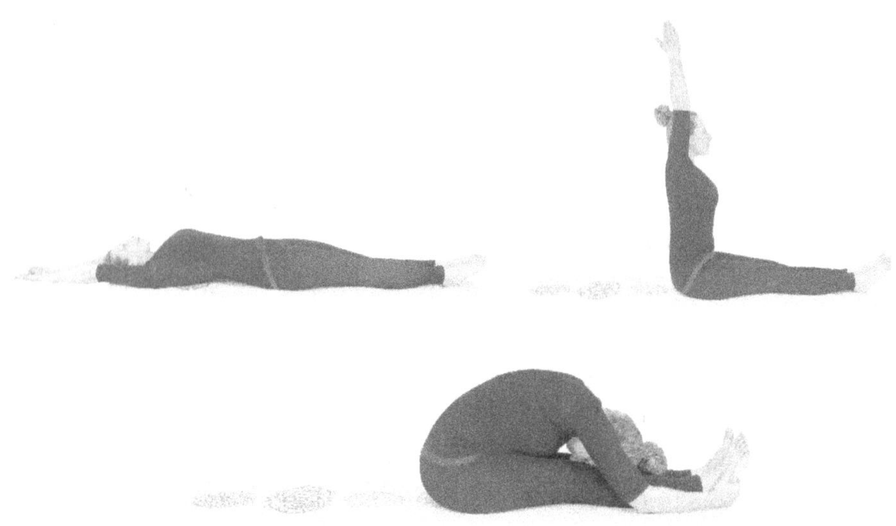

Lie down in a supine position, place your arms overhead and bring them straight to the floor with your palms facing the sky. This is the starting position. Take a moment to relax your body.

**Variation A:**

When you are ready, inhale and while exhaling raise your trunk to a sitting position by engaging your abdominal muscles. Stretch your spine by raising your arms above your head in an attempt to reach for the ceiling. Keep your abdominal muscles engaged. Feel the stretch below your shoulder blades and the rib cage. Feel the tension in the upper arms.

**Variation B:**

When you are ready, inhale and as you exhale raise your trunk slowly to a sitting position by engaging your abdominal muscles. Stretch your spine by raising your arms above your head and smoothly bend forward into the back stretching pose or forward bend or Paschimottanasana.

Here you can retain your breath while holding the position for a short time before returning to the sitting position. Stay for 1-2 breaths in the final position with deep and smooth breathing to stretch your back and hamstrings. Inhale and return slowly to the sitting position by maintaining the position of the arms. Keep them straight above the head and slowly lean backwards to return to starting position. The trunk raise on both the forward and backward bend should be from the hips and by engaging the core. Ensure that you keep your lower back totally relaxed during the practice. This is 1 round. Repeat up to 5-10 times or more.

**Breathing:** Traditionally, in this asana, you must inhale and come to the sitting position, exhale to bend forward, inhale to sit up, and exhale to return to starting position. However, if you would like to strengthen your abdominal area, then practice as described below. Inhale at starting position, exhale to raise your trunk and bend forward to Paschimottanasana, and inhale to return to your starting position slowly.

**Awareness:** Sacral Chakra (Swadhisthana).

**Benefits:** Similar to Paschimottanasana but at a lower impact. This is a dynamic asana which prompts blood circulation and metabolism in the body. It also strengthens the abdominal muscles, promotes flexibility of the body and stimulates physical and pranic energy.

**Precautions:** Similar to Paschimottanasana. Since this is a dynamic asana, people with high blood pressure, heart or back conditions should not practice it.

# Exercise 81:   Inverted pose or Vipareeta Karani Asana

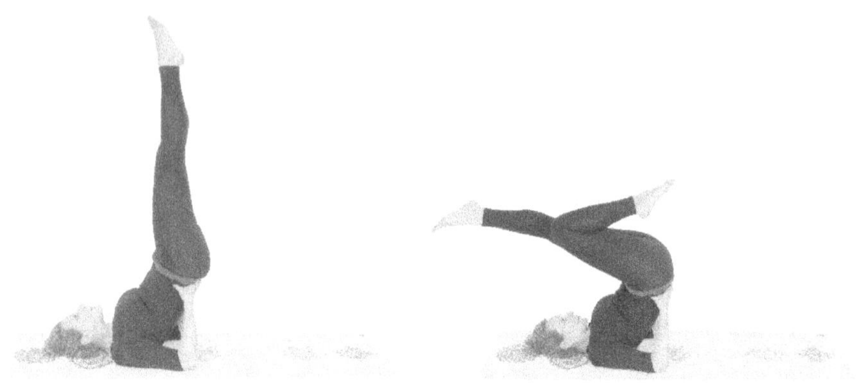

Lie down flat on the ground, and keep your legs straight and your feet together. Place your hands and arms close to your body with the palms facing the ground. Relax your body and take a few deep breaths. When you are ready, inhale and raise your legs and feet together over your body towards the head, using the abdominal muscles. Raise your buttocks and place your palms on top of your hips to help your hands and arms lift your body to raise your legs to a vertical position on the ground. From there, roll your spine from the ground to take your legs further up. In the final position, be aware that your body weight should rest on the shoulders, neck and elbows, the trunk is at 45° angle to the ground, the legs are vertical to the ground and the chin is relaxed. Cup your hips with your palms (and wrists) and maintain position of the legs for as long as it feels comfortable with your eyes closed and your feet relaxed.

To release the pose, lower the legs over the head either together or one by one by bending the knees. Then slowly release your hands and arms, and place them close to your body with your palms facing down. Slowly lower your spine to the ground and feel the motion of each vertebra. Keep your head relaxed on the ground at all times. After your buttocks are on the ground, lower the legs while keeping them straight. Relax in Shavasana until your heart rate and breathing is back to normal. Practice the sequence only once while retaining the final position for the maximum time possible.

**Breathing:** Breathe softly and normally at the final pose. Hold your breath while reaching the final position and while lowering your body to the ground.

**Awareness:** Throat Chakra (Vishuddhi).

**Benefits:** Stimulates the thyroid gland and balances the endocrine, reproductive, nervous, circulatory, digestive and respiratory systems. It also calms the mind and relieves stress and anxiety, boosts the immune system, maintains the good health of the bones, strengthens the legs, abdomen and reproductive organs and tones the nerves passing through the neck to the brain. Blood circulation is increased in the head to rejuvenate the ears, eyes and tonsils. It also revives the skin cells and tissue for a healthier, glowing look.

**Precautions:** Not to be practised by those with enlarged thyroid, liver or spleen, suffering from spondylitis, slipped disk, high blood pressure or other heart conditions, weak blood vessels in the eyes, thrombosis or impure blood. It should be avoided during menstruation and after the 2nd trimester.

**Note:** A common modification for Vipareeta Karani Asana is this one of the legs up the wall. This asana is similar to Sarvangasana, with less pressure on the neck. It is usually practised before or after Halasana, and after Matsyasana, Ushtrasana or Supta Vajrasana.

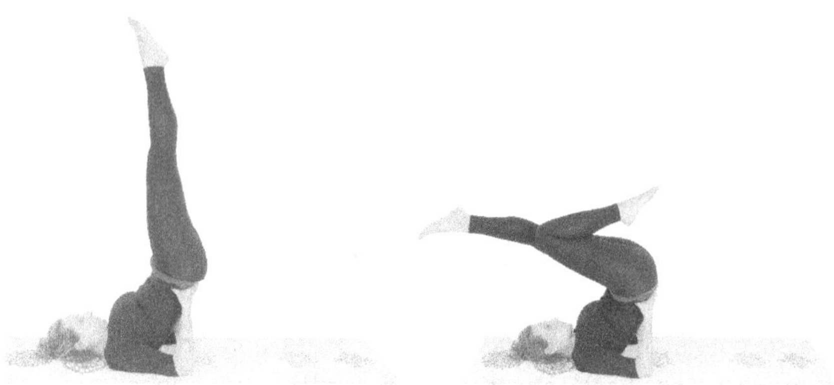

This asana is very similar to the inverted pose or Vipareeta Karani Asana. The difference in practising Sarvangasana lies in two parts:

- the hands are positioned behind the ribcage to hold the position or on the waist,

- the chin is locked to the chest

**Variation:**

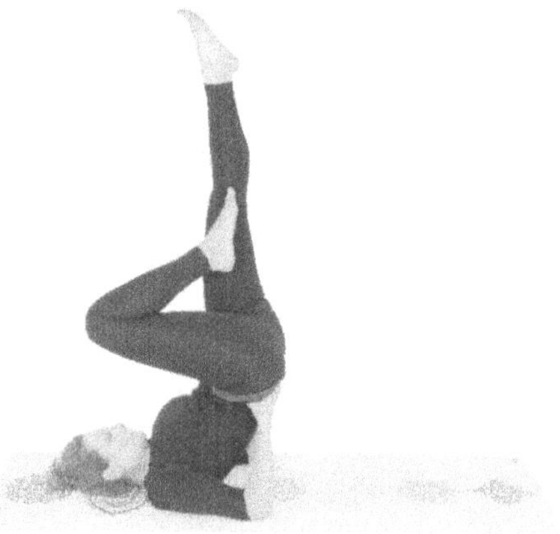

Inhale and bend your right knee and bring your foot to the left knee or its side. For more advanced practitioners, exhale and bend from the hips toward your head, and place the right knee on the forehead. Here, the left leg follows the motion and stays horizontal to the ground. Hold your breath while holding the position. Return to Sarvangasana. Maintain your balance and repeat with the other leg.

**Details:** Same as the inverted pose or Vipareeta Karani Asana.

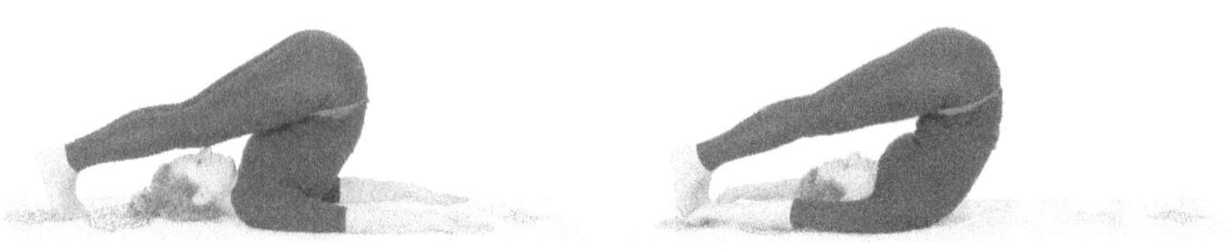

From a supine position, keep your legs straight and feet together. Place your hands and arms close to your body with the palms facing the ground. Relax your body and take a few deep breaths.

When you are ready, inhale and raise your legs and feet together over your body towards the head to come to Sarvangasana. Raise your buttocks and place your palms on top of your hips to help with your hands and arms. The legs are raised to a vertical position compared to the ground. From there, slowly roll your back away from the ground to lower both your legs together over your head. Engage your abdominal muscles to maintain your balance. Aim to touch the floor with your toes. Turn your palms to face the sky, bend your elbows and place your palms behind your ribcage to support your back. You can practice any of the variations given below.

Hold the pose for 30 seconds and gradually add more time to your practice, until you can easily hold it for at least 1 minute. Advanced practitioners can hold the final position for up to 10 minutes or longer.

To release the pose, first lower your arms with your palms facing the ground and as in Vipareeta Karani Asana, gradually lower your spine to the ground, and feel the motion of the vertebrae one after another. Then lower your buttocks and maintain the vertical position of the legs. Engage your abdominal muscles to lower your legs to the starting position, while keeping your knees straight.

**Variation A:**

After balancing on the position you can remove your hands from beside your body and keep them straightened and flat on the ground with the palm facing the ground.

**Variation B:**

On the final position, walk on your toes further away from the head and with your chin locked to your chest, completely stretch your body. Remain in this final position with normal breathing for as long as it feels comfortable.

**Variation C:**

On the final position, walk on your toes further away from the head. Keep the legs straight together. Hold on to the toes with your arms straight. Remain in this final position with normal breathing for as long as this feels comfortable.

**Breathing:** Normal and soft breathing at the final pose. Hold your breath to come into the final position and lower your body to the ground.

**Awareness:** Throat Chakra (Vishuddhi) or Solar Plexus Chakra (Manipura).

**Benefits:** Massages all the internal organs with the diaphragm movement. It stimulates the digestive system and can relieve constipation and dyspepsia, stimulates the spleen and the suprarenal glands, promotes insulin production by the pancreas, improves liver and kidney function, and strengthens the abdominal muscles. It also relieves the back muscles and tones the spinal nerves. It regulates and activates the thyroid gland, balances your metabolism and improves the immune system. Blood circulation is increased to the whole body and the head leading to a healthier-looking face.

**Precautions:** Those who suffer from hernia, slipped disk, sciatica, high blood pressure, back conditions or arthritis of the neck should avoid this asana.

**Counterpose:** Matsyasana, Ushtrasana or Supta Vajrasana

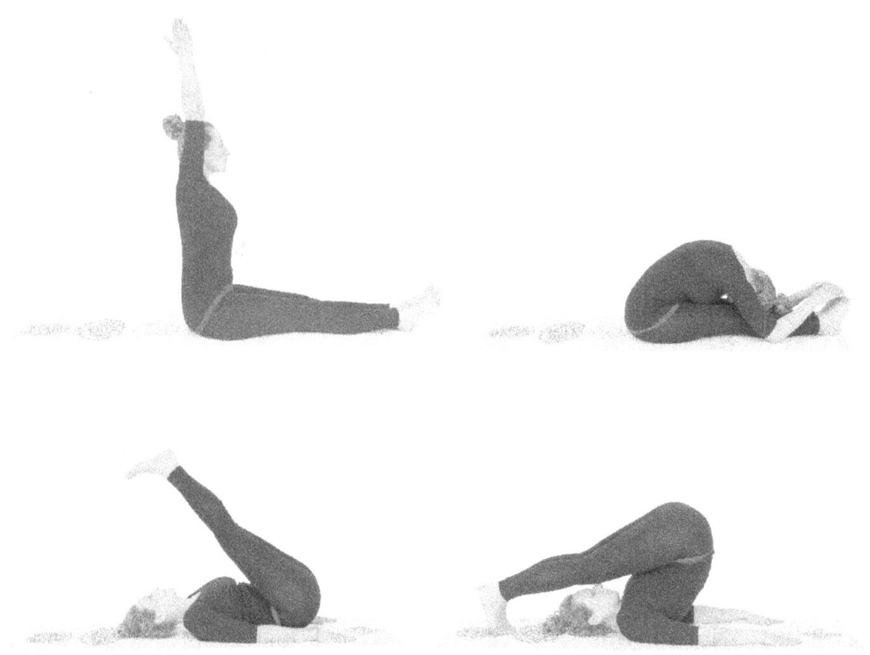

This dynamic asana is a combination of Gatyatmak Paschimottanasana, Sarvangasana and Halasana.

Begin with the supine position and then go to Halasana and hold the position for 1 or 2 breaths. Roll your body back to the supine position and immediately sit up to Paschimottanasana. Hold the position for 1 or 2 breaths. Come to the sitting position to complete 1 round. Practice with a balanced and flowing motion. Repeat 5-10 times.

**Awareness:** Sacral (Swadhisthana) Chakra or Solar Plexus (Manipura) Chakra.

**Counterpose:** Matsyasana or Supta Vajrasana.

**Benefits, Precautions, etc.:** Same as Gatyatmak Paschimottanasana and Halasana.

# Face Massage

Facial massage has many benefits for the head and skin. It relaxes the tension and lessens the expression lines on the face. With increased blood circulation to the facial tissue, your skin can be repaired and rejuvenated and you can look brighter and younger. The massage also stimulates collagen production, softens the wrinkles and smile lines, and firms and tightens the skin. It can lift and make the eyebrows symmetrical. It also improves the looks of the area around the neck and provides a better contour for the face. Any lymphatic drainage will be stimulated and the toxins will be removed from cells, reducing puffiness and inflammation. A face massage is recommended in the morning to remove puffiness. It also tones the muscles and lifts the skin. Moreover, it massages the facial nerve which is connected to the brain, relaxes your mind and relieves you from migraines, insomnia, stress and anxiety.

However, it is not advisable to have a massage more than twice a month, the frequency of which depends solely on your age and skin type. For normal skin, the massage can be done for a maximum of two days per month or once every 3 weeks. For dry skin, it can be done weekly once. For oily skin, massage is not advisable since it may increase the appearance of pimples. But if you do massage, use a moisturizer specific for oily skin.

Face yoga and face massage can prevent the formation of acne and pimples, but if you have oily skin with pimples or acne-prone skin, it is highly recommended that you use a toner before and after face massage to remove any oil or sebum produced naturally overnight. The toner will also help your pores unclog, close and tighten.

If you have open wounds, pimples, acne, eczema or other facial skin conditions, first consult your dermatologist and then massage your face or body. If you still want to do a facial massage in spite of acne or any facial conditions, massage only the parts that are not affected with extra caution.

To perform any type of massage you need 1 or 2 tablespoons of a liquid lubricant, which is usually a carrier oil such as olive oil, coconut oil, almond oil, grapeseed or jojoba oil. In addition to a carrier oil, you may use your moisturizer to help the product penetrate your skin and cells. Using your moisturizer for massaging will act more efficiently on your skin since it is tailored to your skin's specific needs. You may need to reapply it when required so that your skin does not feel stretched while doing the massage.

The hand moves you use while performing the massage can be also practised as an exercise for specific areas. If, for example, you want to work on lifting your eyes, you can isolate those moves and practise these in the form of exercise daily for a maximum of 5 repetitions while you apply your moisturizer.

The pressure applied will depend on your capacity. Since you are massaging your sensitive facial skin, you need not apply too much pressure to avoid overstretching. Overstretching can lead to more lines and wrinkles.

**Reduces signs of ageing:** It helps lighten the appearance of expression lines and wrinkles to make your skin look youthful.

**Pushes toxins out:** You are not only increasing blood circulation but you are also stimulating lymphatic drainage.

**Offers relief from sinus congestion:** With a face massage, the mucus collected in the sinuses can break up to ease pain and allow better breathing.

**Provides glowing skin:** A face massage can turn fatigued skin into a radiant one.

**Improves crepey skin:** A face massage cannot entirely reverse crepey skin. However, it can be combined with other solutions to make the skin firmer and smoother.

**Allows product penetration into the skin:** Your skin products work more efficiently when you massage them into your skin.

**Reduces puffiness:** A face massage can push excessive fluid from our face back to our bloodstream.

**Aids tired eyes:** A cold compress or sliced cucumber or banana peel can reduce puffiness around the eyes. Ice or cold spoons can also work as an alternative. It can also work as a total face toner.

**Promotes relaxation:** Any type of self-care is beneficial for our skin. Our skin will respond to anything we offer to it. Take the time to de-stress by massaging your face, and your skin will show its glow again.

# Positioning of the Arms and Hand Gestures

It is always best to massage your face and practise face yoga exercises in front of a mirror, so that you can see your reflection and moves. In that manner, you can correct the symmetry of your strokes and work on the ideal outcome for your face.

Keep your hands at shoulder level. In this position, you will unintentionally keep your spine erect, correct your body posture and stretch the whole vertebral column. You will also keep the chest open to allow more oxygen into your organs and skin. Most importantly, you will not strain your neck during the massage.

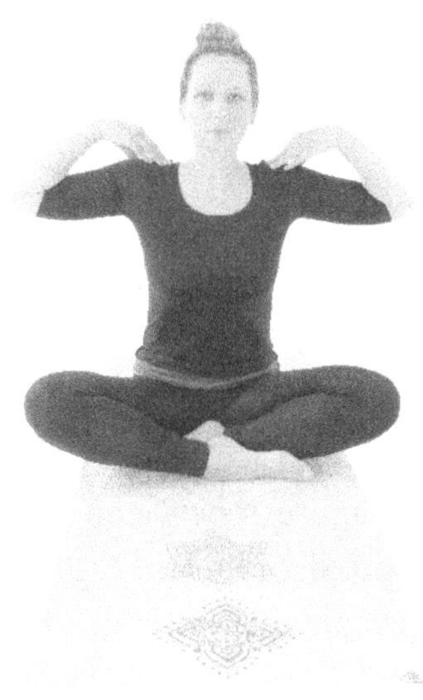

If you plan on doing a full massage, you may require some time in this position. You can take a short break to shake your arms and shoulders and continue. It is recommended that you do some of the warm-up exercises before you start, and some after you finish to not only nourish your skin but also your body and internal organs.

The hand gestures you can use are:

Open palms to caress your skin with less pressure.

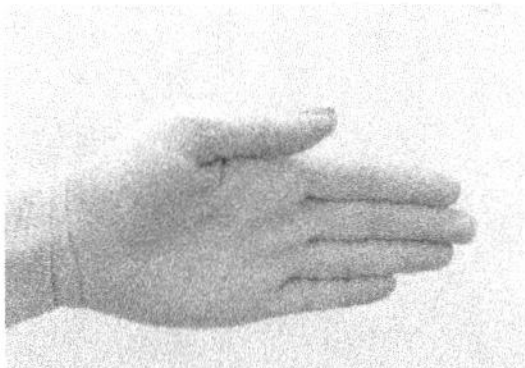

Make a V-shape with your index and middle fingers to stretch your skin with medium pressure. The open palms and the V-shape are ideal, especially for younger skin, and those who have had Botox therapy.

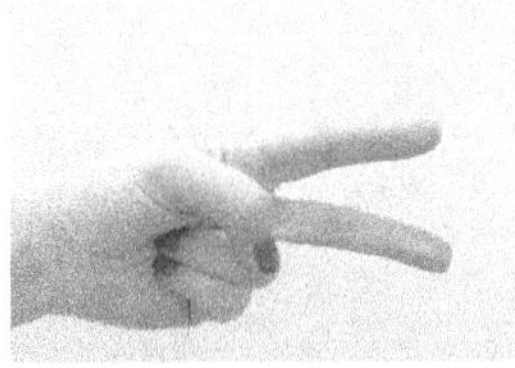

Make a two-finger knuckle shape with your index and middle fingers to apply more pressure. This is ideal for older skin since the extra tension can help reduce wrinkles and lift sagging skin.

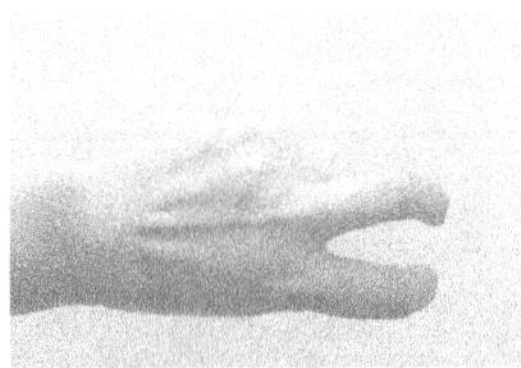

Make a fist knuckle shape for the forehead area or much older skins with controlled pressure to help in lifting the skin and stubborn wrinkles.

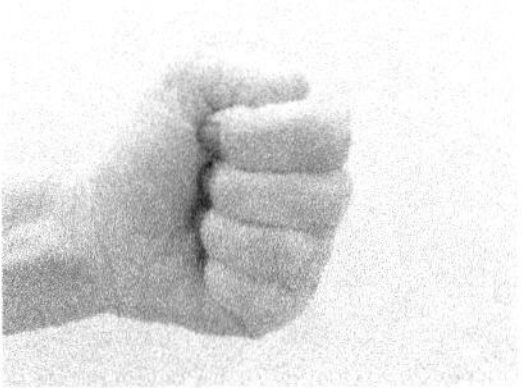

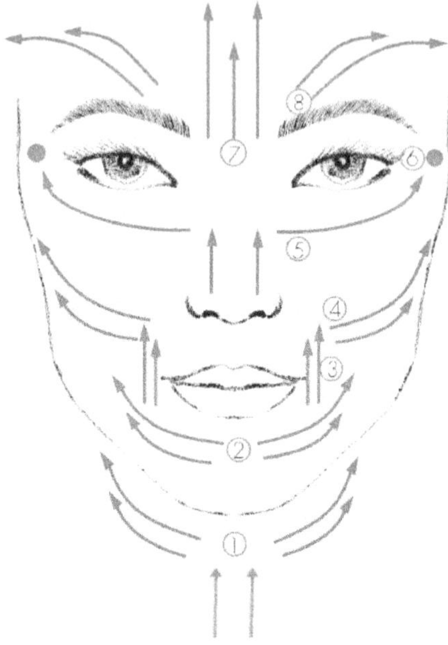

As a principle, we always start from the neck area following the order of strokes to complete each of the face:

1. Neck

2. Jaw

3. Mouth and Lips

4. Cheeks

5. Nose

6. Eyes and Eyebrows

7. Eyebrows Center

8. Forehead and Hairline

9. Ears

If you would like to add some aroma to your massage, essential oils can be used. However, essential oils are very strong and you should never use them on the whole face or skin in their original form. They come in such small bottles because the amount needed is just one drop or less for direct use. Those having acne can consult their dermatologist before using an essential oil. The application of essential oil is just 1 drop or less on the fingertip and if placed on the pimple, it will help it dry out.

There are many essential oils available on the market. You can choose to use T3, peppermint, rosemary, or any other that you have used previously and has worked for your skin type.

An old remedy to dry a pimple is to put a cotton ball in hot water, squeeze all the excess water out and use the steam on the spot to clean the bacteria in that particular area. If you want to do the same with another pimple, you will need a new cotton ball to repeat the process. If the pimple is not a stubborn one, after 2-3 days it will start drying out. Just remember not to touch it with your hands or nails, as tempting as it may be.

So, essential oils are to be used directly only on a pimple and in acne only after consulting your dermatologist. If you want to massage them into your face or in any other area of your body, 1-2 drops mixed with 10-15 ml of carrier oil are needed. The most common carrier oils are olive oil, coconut oil, almond oil, grapeseed and jojoba. Mustard oil and sesame oil are mostly cooking oils and should not be used for a massage under any circumstances. These are hot oils and might cause allergies or skin irritation or create black marks on the skin.

If you have acne, you cannot use any oil on your face or wherever it develops, because it will increase the moisture in the area that you are trying to dry out. Also, you already have oily skin with acne, so oil is not your solution. Cure your condition first and then massage with oil.

## The Neck

It is important to massage your neck as well. Include the front, sides and back of the neck. Other than the aesthetic part of neck massaging, you need to consider how daily stress contributes to your physique and how it increases tension and pain in the neck. Strokes to the side and back of the neck can relieve pain, tension and stress, whereas frontal strokes lift the skin. So, while you massage your neck, you are indirectly relieving it from all this tension and helping yourself relax mentally. With this relaxation technique, you can reduce your stress levels, migraines, insomnia, anxiety or even anger.

You must always start the face massage from the chest and neck area and move towards the jawline and gradually to the forehead.

## Exercise 85:    Lifting the chest

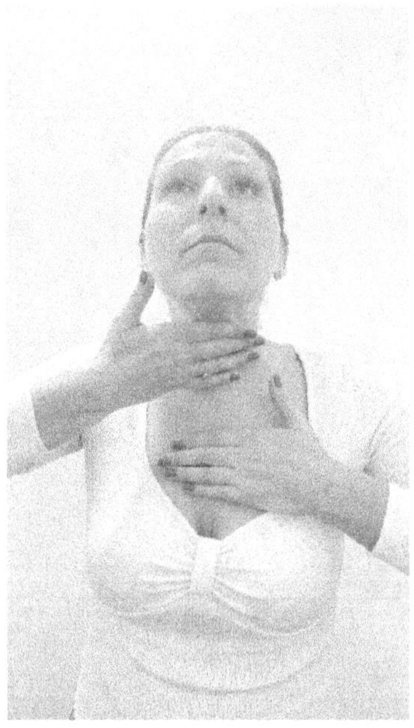

To lift the skin in your chest area, keep your palms open and start your strokes from your chest area to the centre of your neck i.e. the throat. Move your palms one after the other. Do the same on the left and right side of your chest area. Repeat 5-10 times.

**Step 1:**

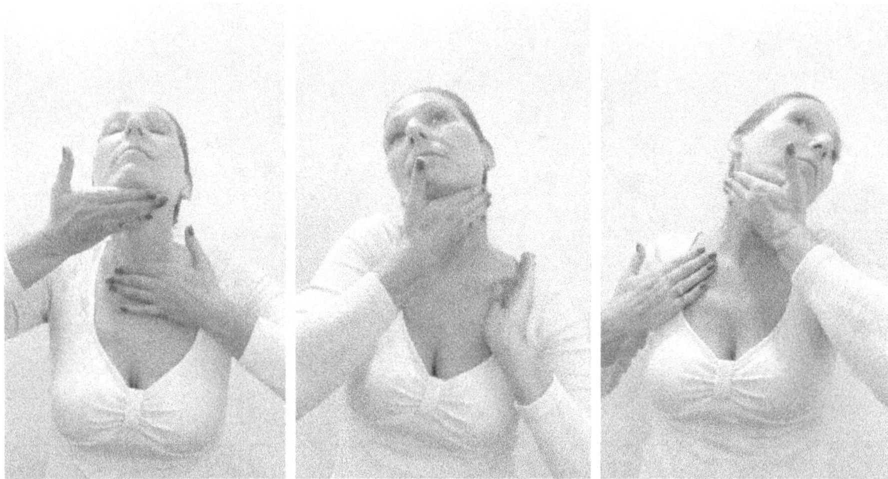

To lift your double chin, start from your collarbone, move to your upper neck, then up to the jaw and the area under the chin. Tilt your head back or to the side to help the motion. Move your palms one after the other. Do the same to the left and right side of your neck while stroking upwards from your collarbone up to your jawbone. Repeat 5-10 times.

**Step 2:**

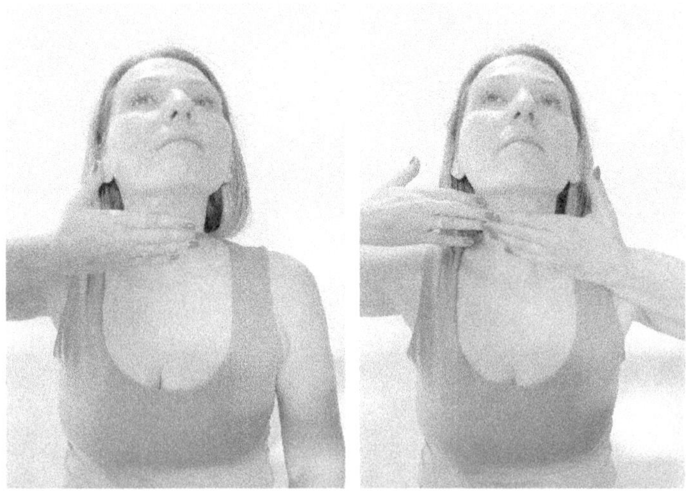

Follows the steps in Step 1, but this time your strokes should be sideways. Repeat 5-10 times.

**Step 3:**

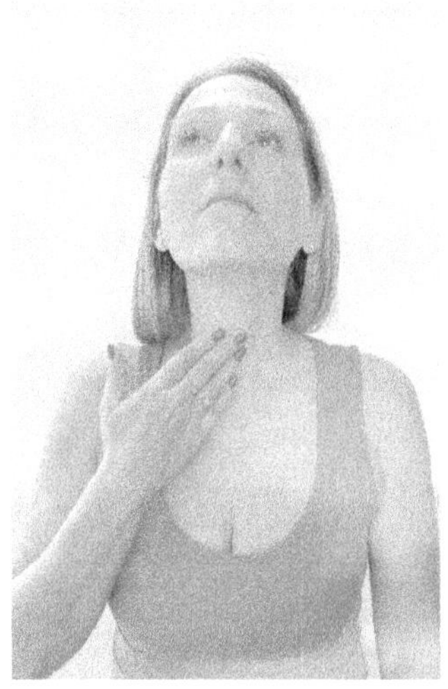

Place your fingers on your throat and perform small circular motions clockwise and anticlockwise. Repeat 5-10 times.

**Step 4:**

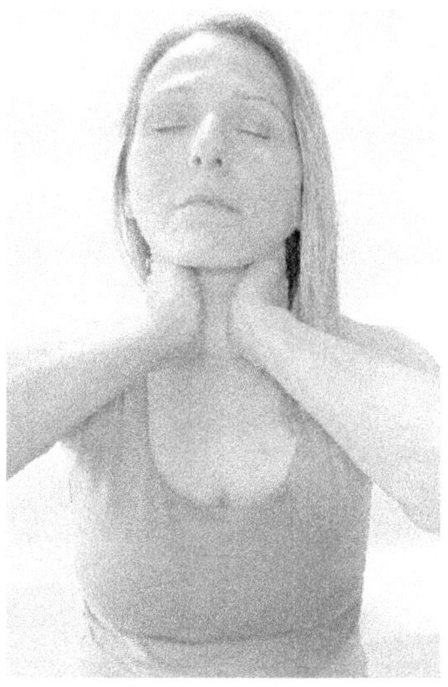

To lift the skin in front of the neck, place your palms open like a pyramid with your fingertips placed just on top of the collarbone. Stroke the skin on the sides and back of the neck up to your hairline. Repeat 5-10 times. Do the same starting from your throat area and repeat an equal amount of times. Do the same starting from the double chin area and repeat an equal amount of times.

# Exercise 87: Lifting the back of the neck

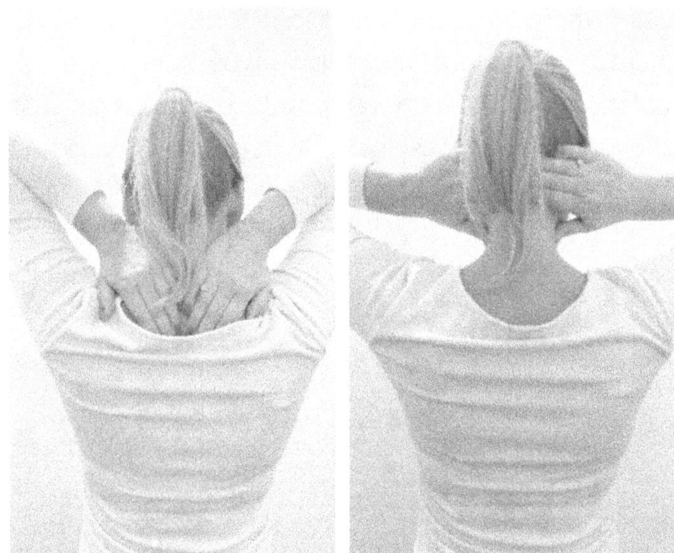

Begin with step 4 outlined in the section on lifting the frontal portion of the neck and move your hands as far down as you can reach past your cervical bone (the top of your vertebrae). From there, swipe your hands up toward the hairline or just below. This is a very relieving and relaxing technique for the back of the neck which also lifts the skin. Repeat 5-10 times.

Relax your shoulders. Take a few deep breaths. Continue with your face.

The main aim when practising a massage for the jawline is to shape it. But its benefits are far more important for your face since the improved blood circulation increases the temperature of muscular tissue which relieves the tight facial muscles and develops the elasticity of the fascia. It can also release the tension in the jaw for clinchers and teeth grinders.

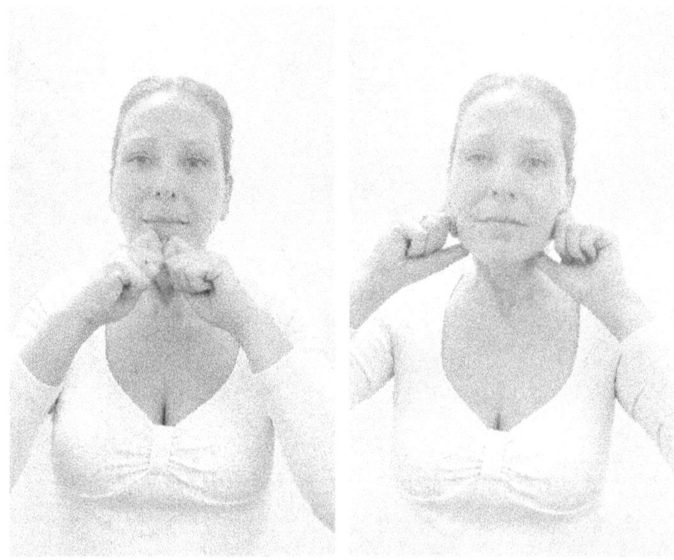

Lift your chin if you want to work harder on the double chin or keep your head straight. Make a two-finger knuckle and place your fingers in the centre of your chin. From there, stroke across your jawline and up to your ears. Repeat 5-10 times.

On the last stroke, maintain the position and bring your knuckles under your ears. Massage the sides of the neck with your thumbs with upward movements only. Repeat 5-10 times.

# Exercise 89:  Shaping the jawline without pressure

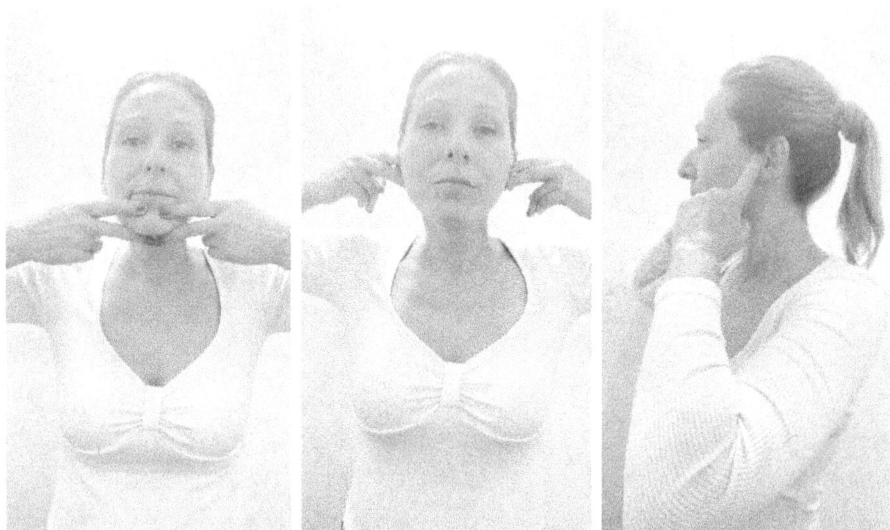

Keep your head straight and place your V-shaped fingers in the middle of your chin. Simultaneously, move both hands to the sides following the jawline to help with lifting the double chin and shaping the jawline. Repeat 5-10 times.

On the last repetition, press the acupressure point in front of the tragus (the middle of your ear) for 3 seconds and release.

With mouth massage, you are not only lifting its corners but also aiming to help blood circulation in that area. Any lymphatic drainage and flow in that area will be released and can relieve tension in the jaw for clinchers and teeth grinders.

There are techniques for intra-oral massage also which are more efficient and effective if someone else is doing it for you. These are not going to be presented in this book. But you can practice the tongue exercises as presented in this chapter for intra-oral massage and health.

In the case of your lips, when you massage them daily, you tone and strengthen them, and also make them look fuller, larger and rosier in the most natural way. Beeswax, paraffin-based lip balms or simple olive/coconut oil are more efficient for moisturization as these will not evaporate quickly and will keep your lips hydrated for longer periods.

**Step 1:**

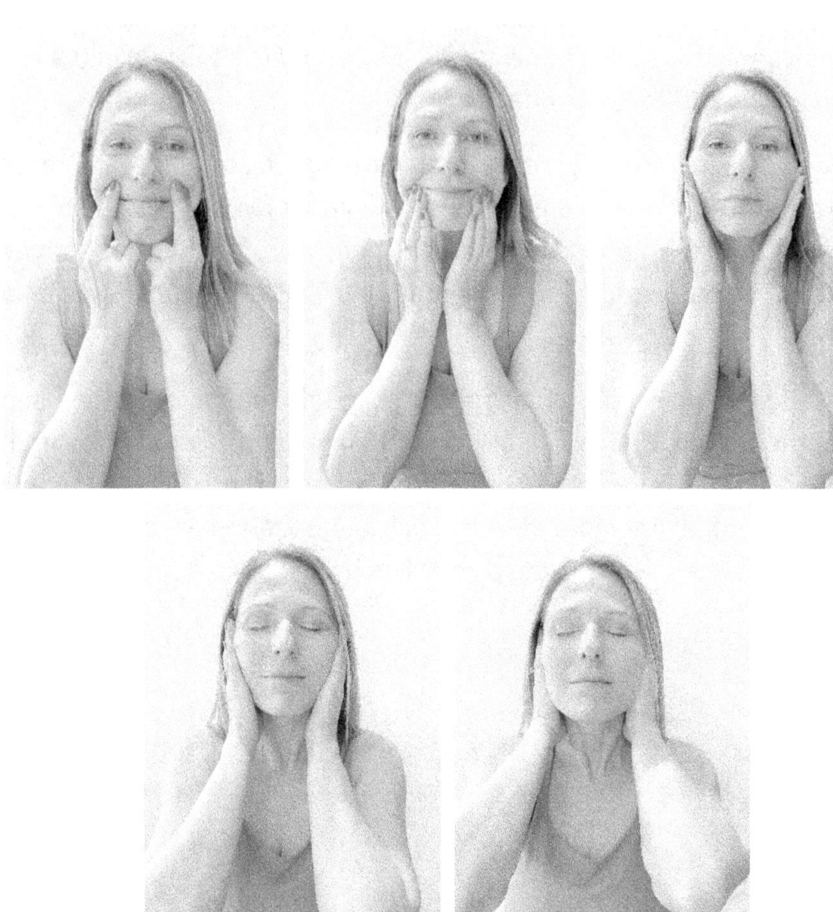

As a warm-up, start applying pressure in circular motions in the area around the mouth on each spot. You can engage 1, 2 or more fingers together during the practice. Repeat 5-10 times.

In the end, gently stretch your skin from the sides of the mouth toward your ears and hold the position for 5-10 seconds.

**Step 2:**

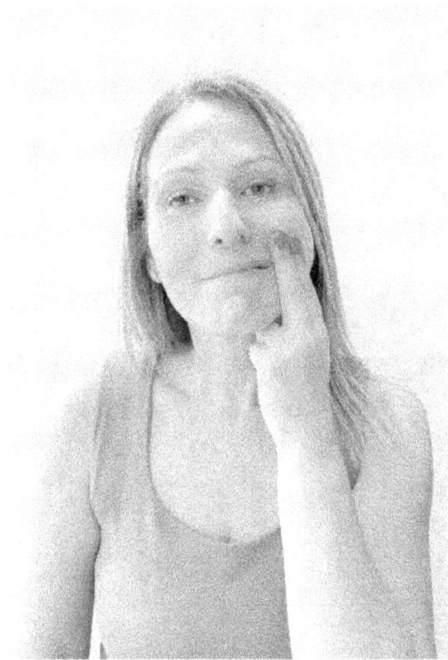

Then lift and hold either both sides together or one side at a time with any hand. Follow the natural motion of your face.

**Step 3:**

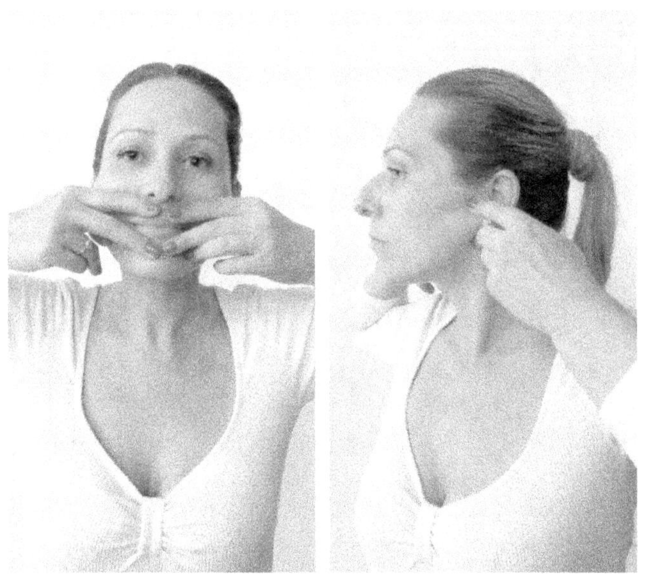

Place your V-shaped fingers around your mouth, with the index fingers above the upper lip and the middle fingers below the lower lip. You can massage with simultaneous motion with your head straight. You can move your hands to the sides and up, following the mouth and below the cheekbones. Or with a gentle movement of the head from right and left and the arms stable in the position. You can maintain a smile to help lift the corners of the mouth better. Repeat 5-10 times.

On the last repetition, press the acupressure point for 3 seconds in front of the tragus-the middle of your ear, and release.

**Note:** You can do the same with two-finger knuckles if you want to work on deeper wrinkles.

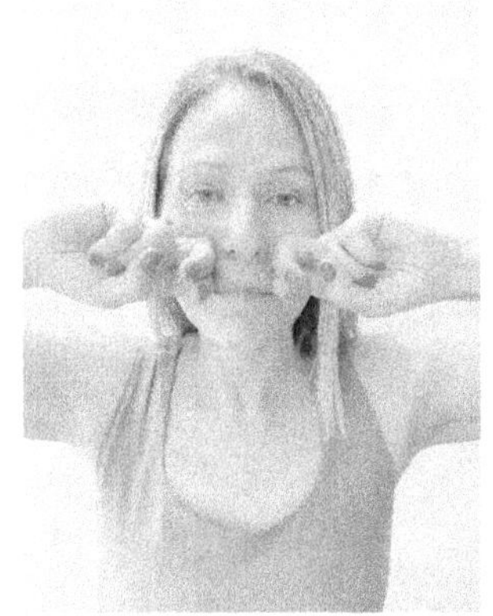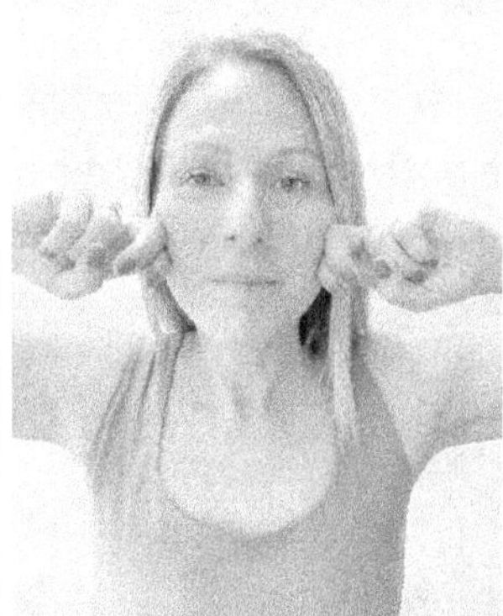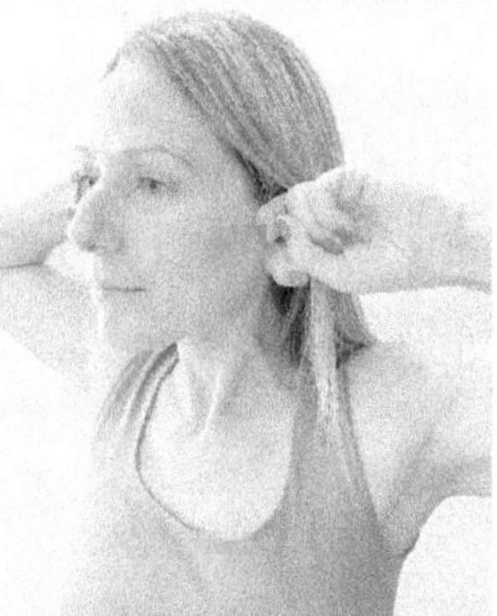

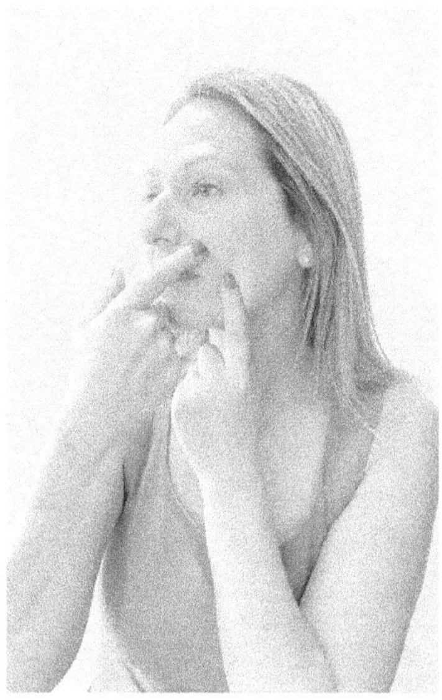

Bend your head slightly to the right. Place your right index finger above the corner of your mouth and your left index finger below it. [You can engage 2 fingers if you need an extra stretch]. Stroke the fingers in opposite directions to stretch the skin that goes diagonally across your denture and through your nasolabial folds. Do this 5-10 times.

**Alternative:** Hold the skin at the lower part of your mouth corners with your left index finger and apply upward strokes with your right index finger.

**Benefits:** Reduces fine lines and wrinkles in the corners of the mouth and smoothens the nasolabial folds.

# Exercise 92:    Massaging the lips

**Step 1:**

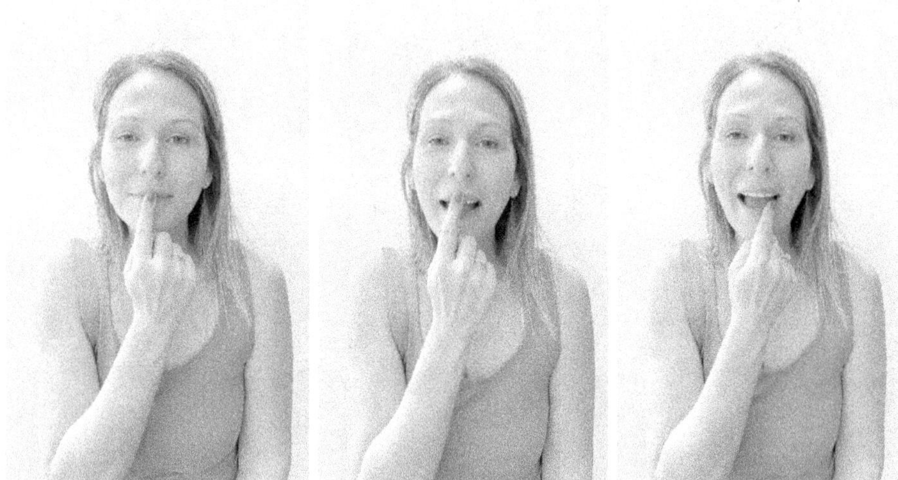

To warm your lips up for the massage, gently press your fingertips into them in every direction. You can open your mouth slightly to help the motion. The warm-up will increase the blood circulation in the area and will relax the muscles underneath. Practice this for 20-30 seconds.

**Step 2:**

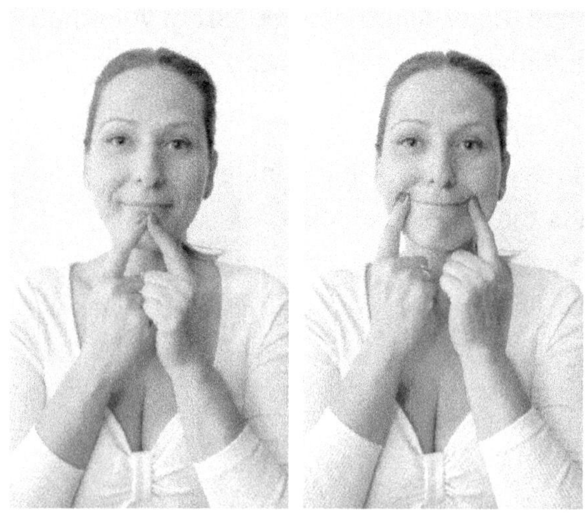

Practice the joker smile exercise, as described in the earlier chapter.

**Step 3:**

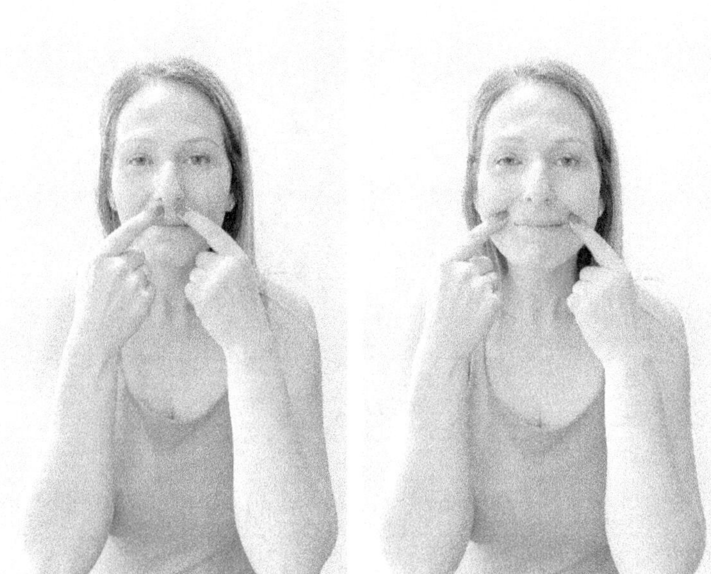

Apply pressure with your fingertips into the area above the lips at the philtrum and start making 5 circular moves in one direction on the spot. Do the same at the sides of the philtrum and across the area above the lip to the corners of the mouth. Focus only on 3-4 points. Repeat 5-10 times.

**Step 4:**

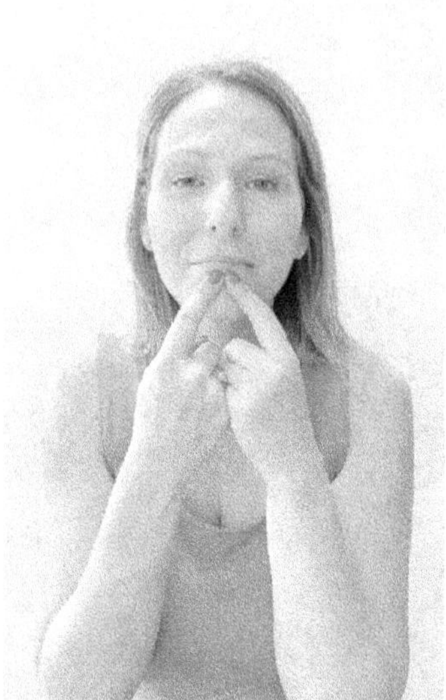

Like in Step 3, do the same at the lower lip, under the lip and across the lip line.

**Benefits:** Tones and strengthens the muscles around your mouth, triggering their growth and making your lips look fuller. Smoothens the lines around the mouth and lips.

# Exercise 93:    Massage for fuller lips

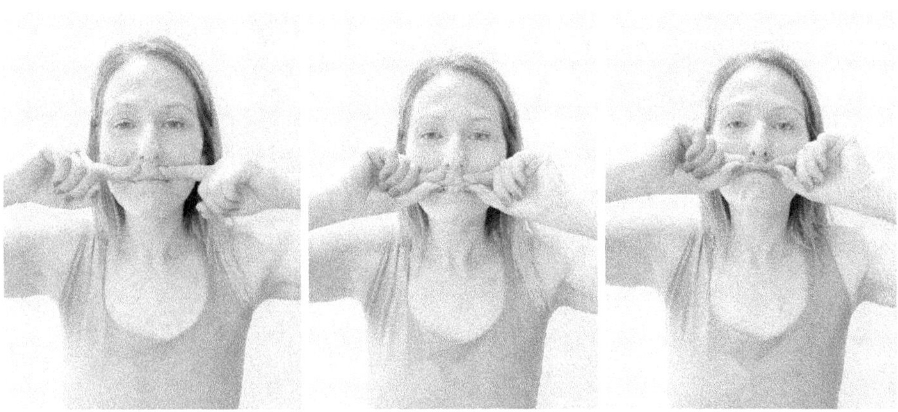

Place your index fingers firmly above your upper lip and using your thumbs try to flip your lip over your index fingers. Hold the position gently for 3 seconds and release. Repeat 5-10 times.

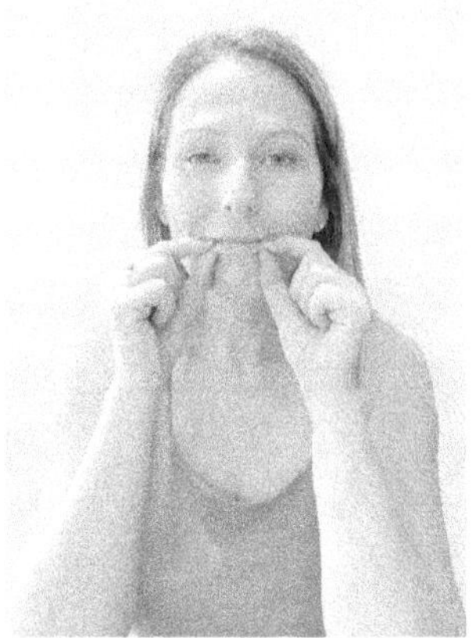

Similarly, place your thumbs firmly below your lower lip and use your index fingers to flip the lip over your thumbs. Hold the position gently for 3 seconds and release. Repeat 5-10 times.

**Benefits:** Tones and strengthens the muscles around your mouth, triggering their growth and making your lips look fuller. You can choose to practice on both your upper and lower lips or any one, according to your needs.

# Exercise 94:    Pinching your lips

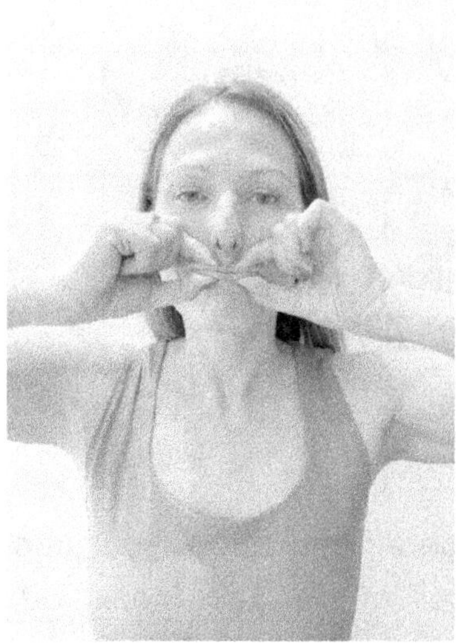

Pout your lips and place your index fingers above the lip and the thumbs below the lip. Press your index fingers down and your thumbs up to pinch the skin. Hold the position for 3 seconds and release. Repeat 5-10 times.

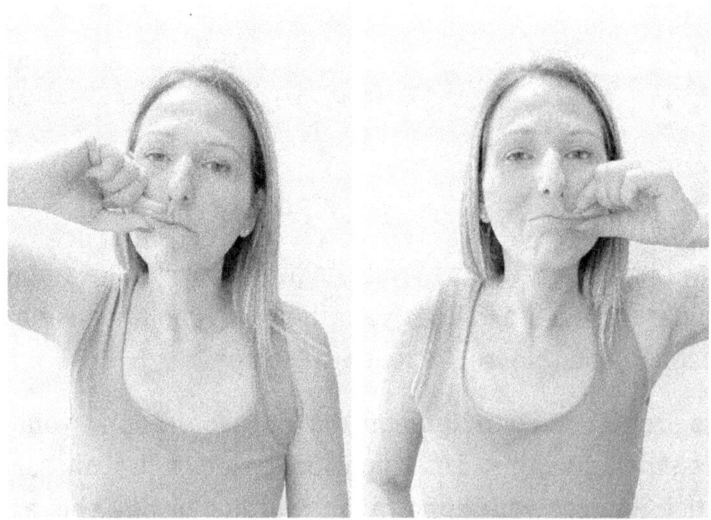

Place your left thumb below the lower lip and the left index finger above the upper lip, pinch and lift it sideways, following the natural motion. With your right index finger hold down the skin from the chin area if you like. Hold the position for 3 seconds and release. Repeat 5-10 times on each side.

**Benefits:** Tones and strengthens the muscles around your mouth, creating more volume on the lips. It also lifts the corners of your mouth.

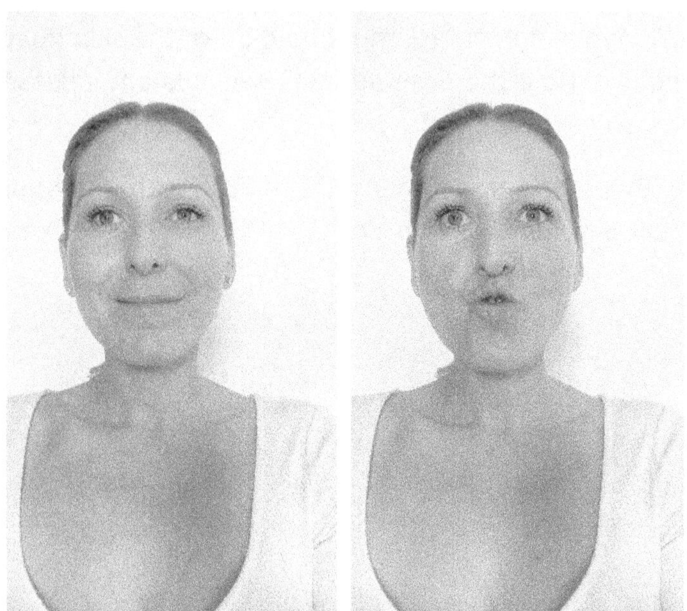

To relax your lips and mouth from previous exercises, do the smile and kiss exercise a few times.

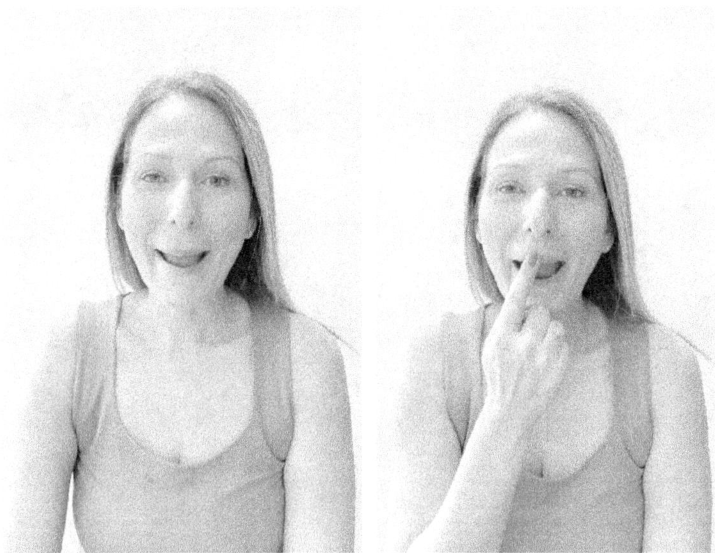

Smile again and curl your lips over your teeth. With any finger, stroke your upper and lower lips an equal amount of times clockwise and anticlockwise. Repeat 5-10 times.

After the last repetition, practice the kiss exercise for 3-5 seconds to relax them.

**Benefits:** Smoothens the lines on and around your lips and relaxes them.

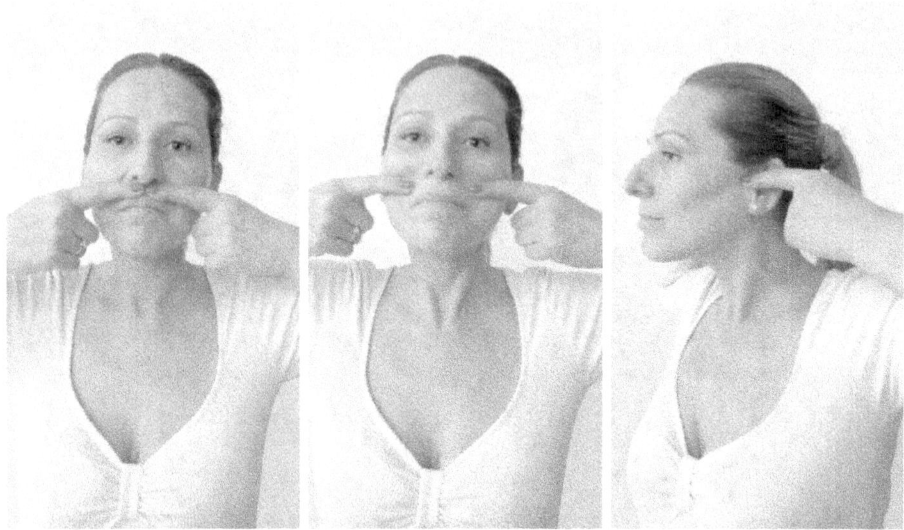

Smile and place your index fingers above the upper lip, starting from the centre to under the nose. You can do the same with a knuckle by applying pressure with the middle finger. While stroking, move your hands to the sides on an upward movement and under the cheekbones. This technique will help in lifting the corners of your mouth and reduce wrinkles in the moustache region and nasolabial folds. Repeat 5-10 times.

On the last repetition, press the acupressure point in front of the tragus-the middle of your ear for 3 seconds and release.

Massaging the nose can help shape it, give it a narrow shape and straighten it. It can also help those who suffer from migraines.

You can use certain techniques to massage the muscles of the nose and a branch of the facial nerve called the buccal nerve. It is responsible for spontaneous eye blinking, moving the nostrils and upper lip and raising the corners of the mouth to smile. Massaging the muscles of the nose and facial nerve innervates many areas of the head and neck region. It also reduces swelling in the nose area and can help with migraines.

If your nose is already slim and narrow, do not practice the nose techniques frequently.

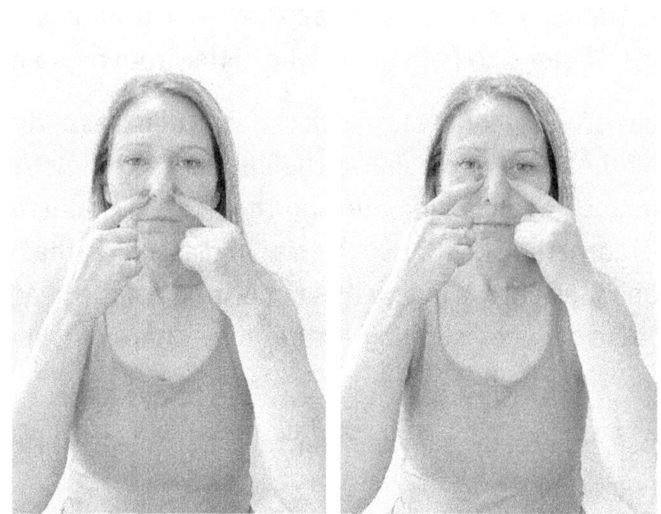

Place your index or middle finger just beside your nostrils, and apply some pressure to make an '8' shape up to the top of the nasal bone. Repeat 5-10 times clockwise and anticlockwise.

After the last repetition, position your fingers just above the nostrils and press with circular moves to massage in one direction for 10-20 seconds. If you have a blocked nose, you can breathe more easily after doing this exercise.

Take a break to inhale and exhale deeply 3-5 times and relax.

# Exercise 99:   Slimmer nostrils

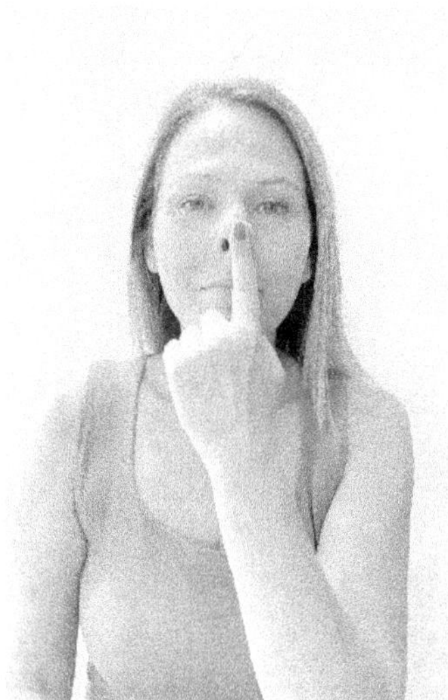

To reduce the size of the tip of your nose and nostrils, smile and place your index finger on the tip of your nose and push it up. Stay for 3-5 seconds on each repeat. Repeat up to 30 times per day.

This technique slims and strengthens the muscles around the nose and reduces wrinkles on the lower part of the nose.

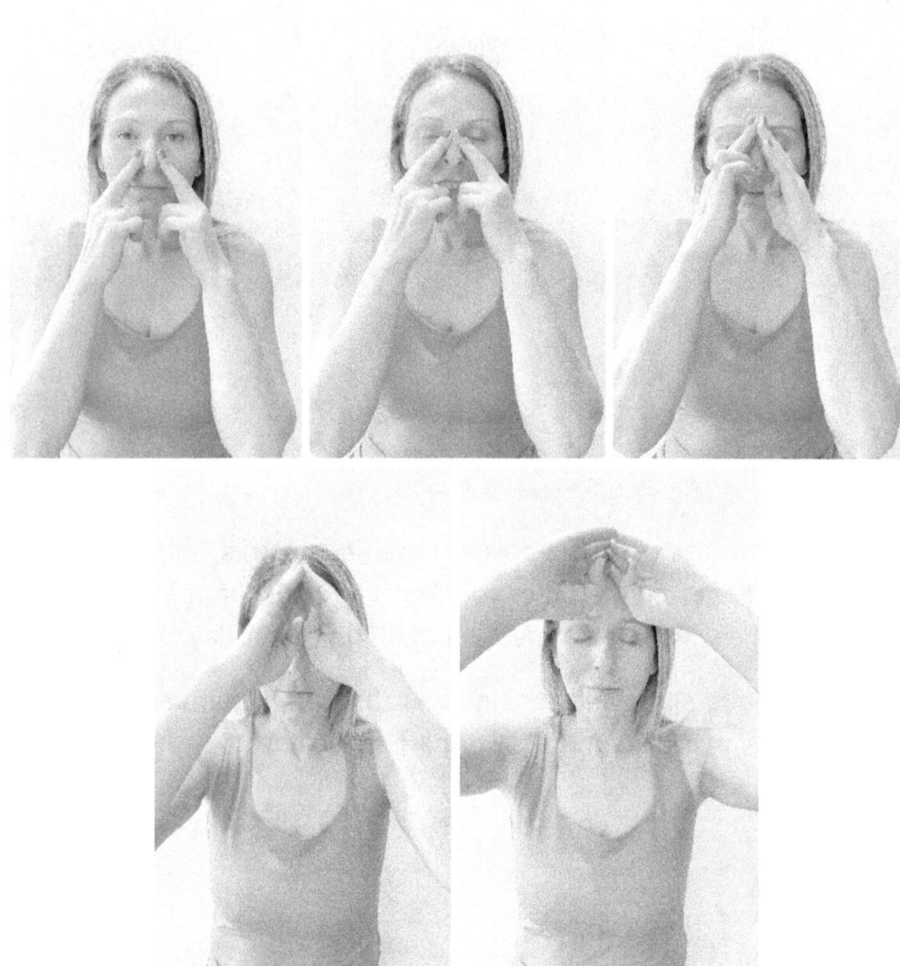

Place your index fingers on the sides of the nostrils and massage with upward movements up to the nose and the centre of your forehead and hairline. With this technique, you will lift your nose. Repeat 5-10 times.

# Exercise 101:   Tip of the nose

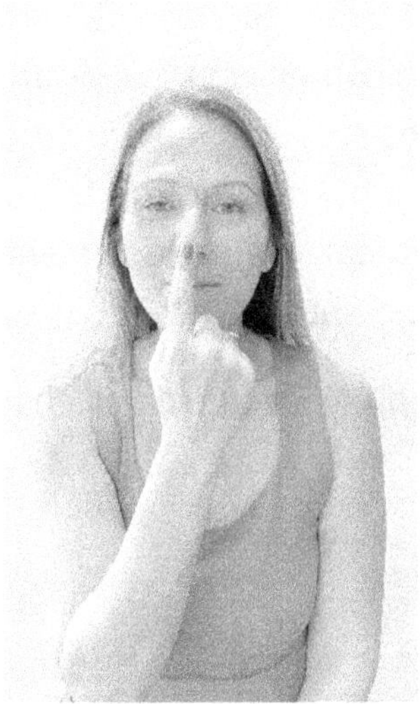

Place any one finger on the tip of your nose to massage it in a circular motion. Repeat at least 20-30 times in one direction only. The next day, choose the other direction.

After a rhinoplasty, there is usually swelling along the sides of the nose and at its tip and this technique helps reduce the swelling after healing. In such conditions, you should practice for at least 2 minutes twice a day and follow your surgeon's instructions.

In normal cases, it makes the tip of the nose shine with a natural blush.

# The Cheeks

Massaging the cheeks increases blood flow to the facial tissue which helps your skin look brighter and younger. Lymphatic drainage is stimulated and the toxins are removed from the cells, reducing swelling and puffiness. Practise it in the morning to remove puffiness. Further, with this technique, you can maintain the shape and pattern of your cheeks and help slim and shape them.

Stroke upwards and begin with the lower cheek before moving to the upper cheek.

# Exercise 102:   Lifting the lower cheeks A

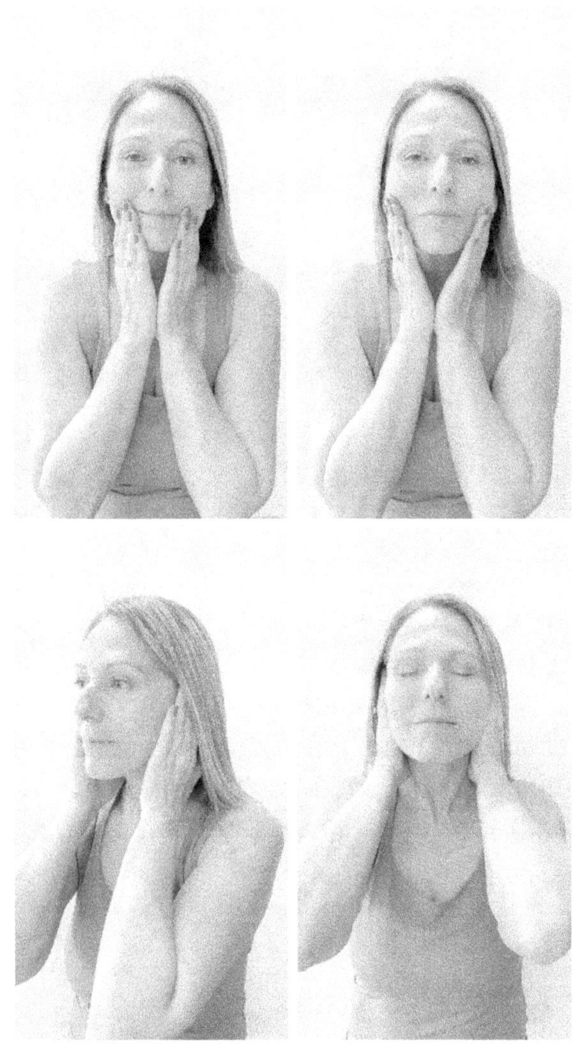

Position your fingers beside your nostrils. Follow the line under the cheekbone with a U-shape stroke up to your ears. Repeat 5-10 times.

On the last repetition, hold the stretch for 5-10 seconds. To maintain the stretch, position your palms with the fingers on the ears and apply extra stretch with your pinky fingers.

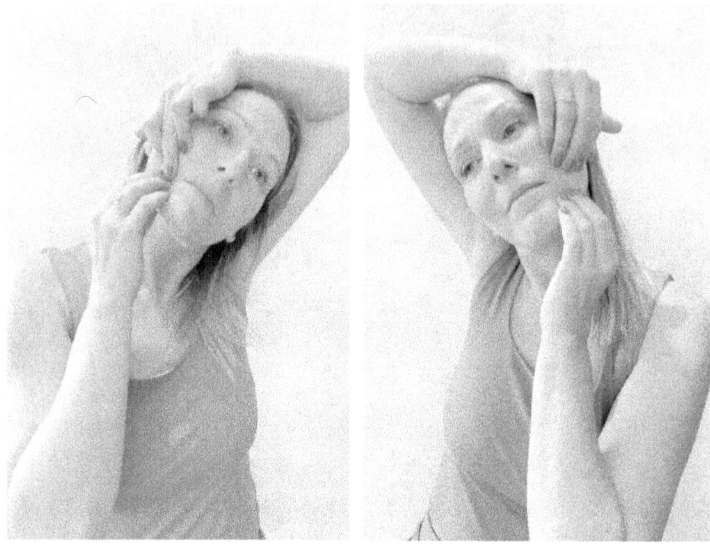

Place the fingers of your left hand beside the left corner of your mouth. Bend your head slightly to the right and bring the right hand over your head so that the fingers of your hand are above the left corner of your mouth. Hold your skin with your left hand and use your right hand to stroke up towards the top of your ear. On the last stroke, keep your skin stretched up to the top of your ear with your right hand. Repeat 5-10 times or more.

## Alternative

If your cheeks are alright or if you want to work less on the cheeks and more on the lines around your mouth and corners of your lips, then practice like above by tapping and stretching your skin at the same time. Or you can do the same with just one hand. Smile while you are doing that. On the last repetition, drag the skin up to the ear and hold the position for 10 seconds. Repeat 5-10 times at least with a continuous motion. Repeat the same with the right side of the face.

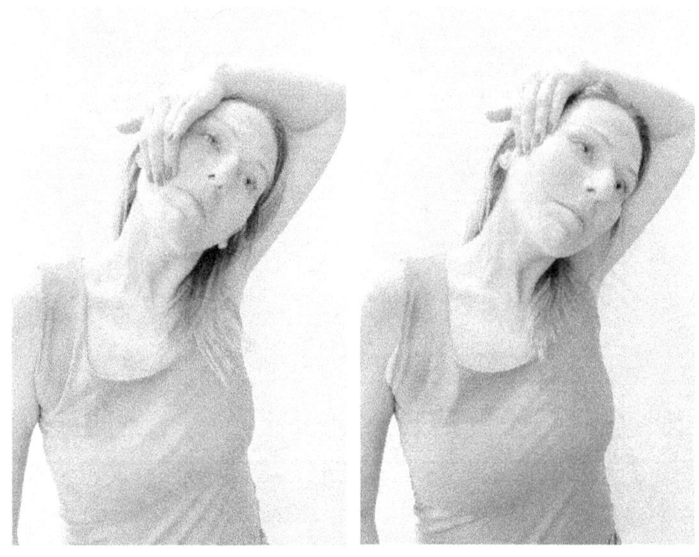

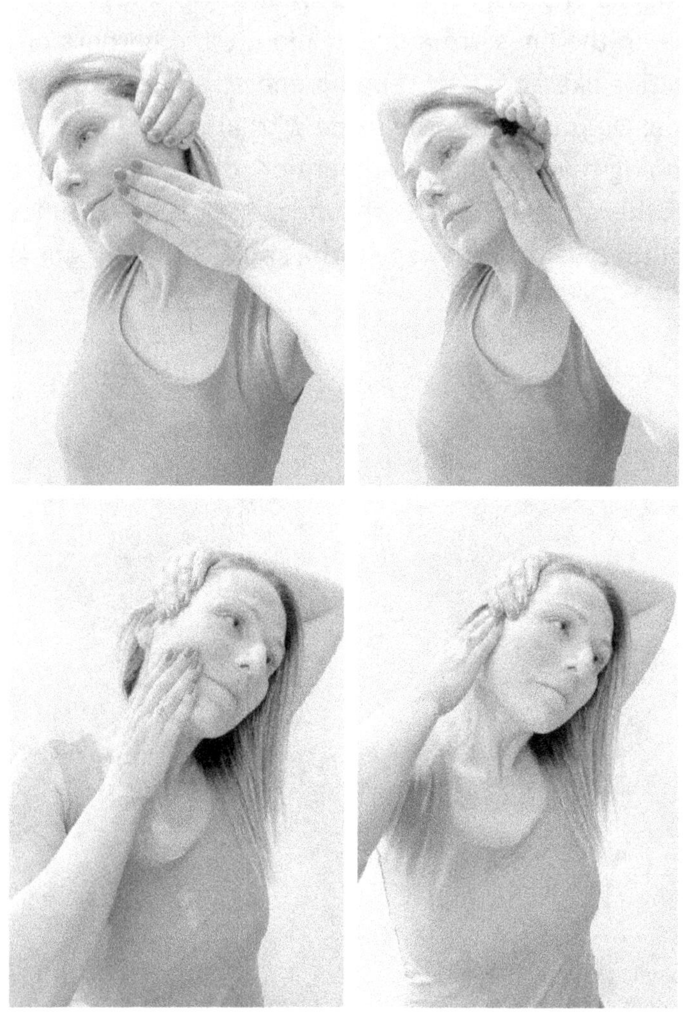

To massage the sides of the cheeks, bend your head to the left and bring your left arm over your head and place it beside the right ear. The thumb should overlap with the ear. With your right palm start the stroke from the top corner of your mouth, drag it up toward the ear, and lift the left palm to hold the stretch for a second. On the last repetition, hold the stretch with both hands together for 10 seconds.

With continuous upward strokes, repeat 5-10 times at least on each side of the face.

**Benefits:** With age, your skin sags and this is how you end up with droopy lips. Practice this daily to lift the cheeks as well as the corners of your mouth.

## Exercise 105:   Lifting of upper cheeks

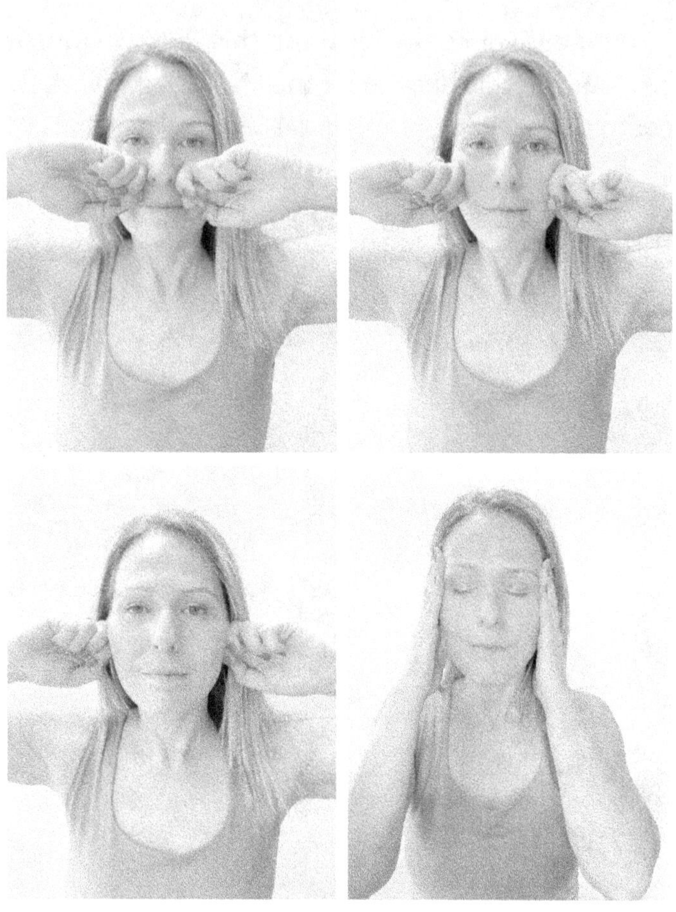

For the upper cheeks, make a knuckle with your index finger and start stroking from under the eye bone and beside the top of the nose. Your middle finger should follow the stroke under the cheekbone. With a U-shape motion, stroke to the side of your face toward the upper side of the ears up to your temples. Be careful about your eyes during the strokes. On the last repetition, stroke to the temples and apply some pressure for 3-5 seconds. Repeat 5-10 times.

Afterwards, hold your skin with your fingers stretching the areas of upper cheeks to eyebrows for 5-10 seconds.

# Exercise 106:   Relaxation of the cheeks

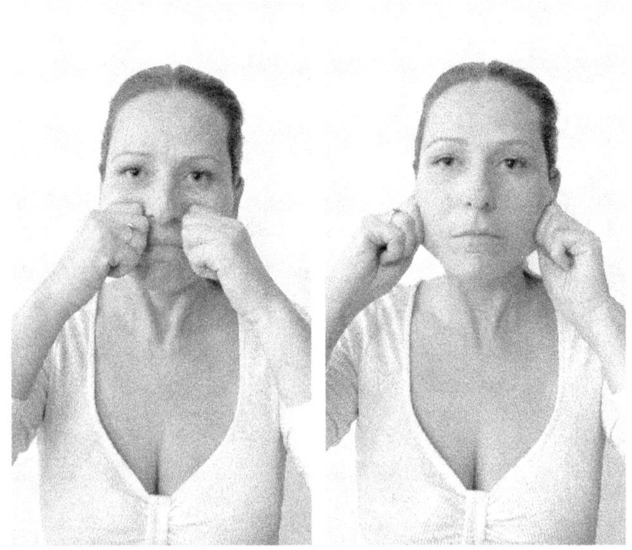

Pinch your cheeks gently, starting from the area beside your nostrils. Start pinching toward the centre of your cheeks and to the ears. Continue by placing your fingers beside your nose and move gradually to the centre of the cheeks and next to the ears. Breathe normally. Repeat 5-10 times.

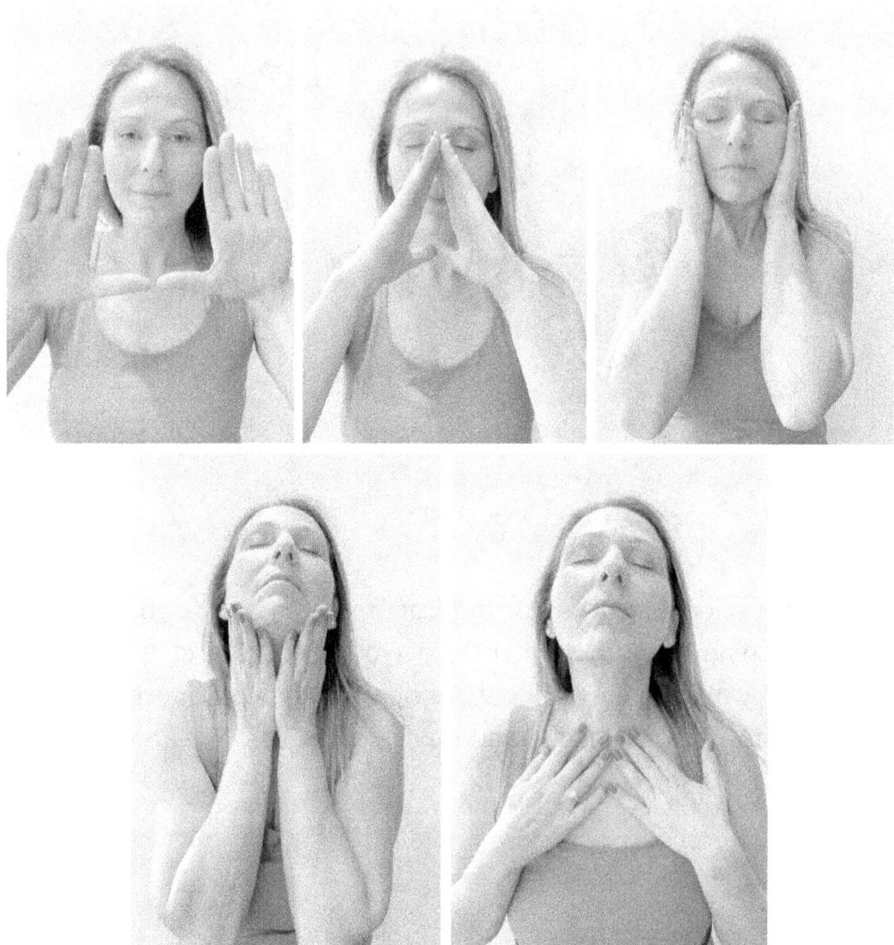

After you are done with your cheek massage, make an L-shape to connect your thumbs and stroke upward from your nose and corners of your mouth to your cheeks and temples. From there, stroke down beside your ears to the sides of your jaw and neck, down to the collar bone and the front of the neck to end the motion on your chest area. Close your eyes and with deep, slow breathing feel the lifting on every part of your face. Repeat 3-5 times if needed.

Face massage around the eyes can support eye health. Headaches can be initiated by eye strain. Eye strain is a common condition in our modern lifestyle and can occur from prolonged screen time or driving, extreme fatigue, insomnia or even from incorrect compatibility of vision and spectacles. Eye strain can lead to headaches and eye massage can relieve you from both. It can also relieve you from dry and tired eyes and reduce puffiness and dark circles.

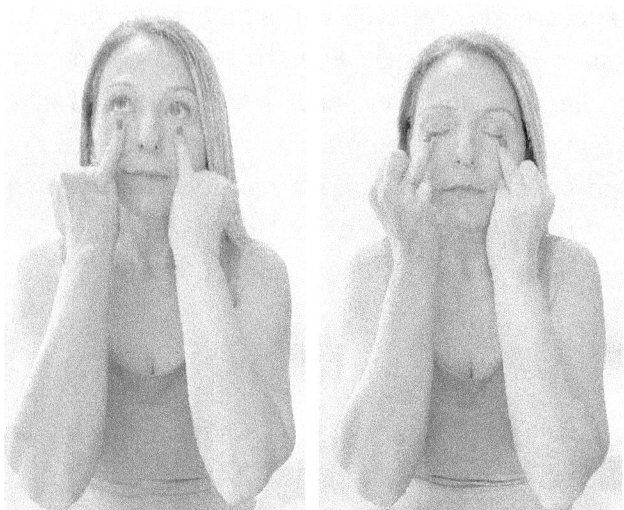

Start with your head in a neutral position, gaze up and tap gently below your eyes with one finger. If gazing up gives you vertigo, you can close your eyes.

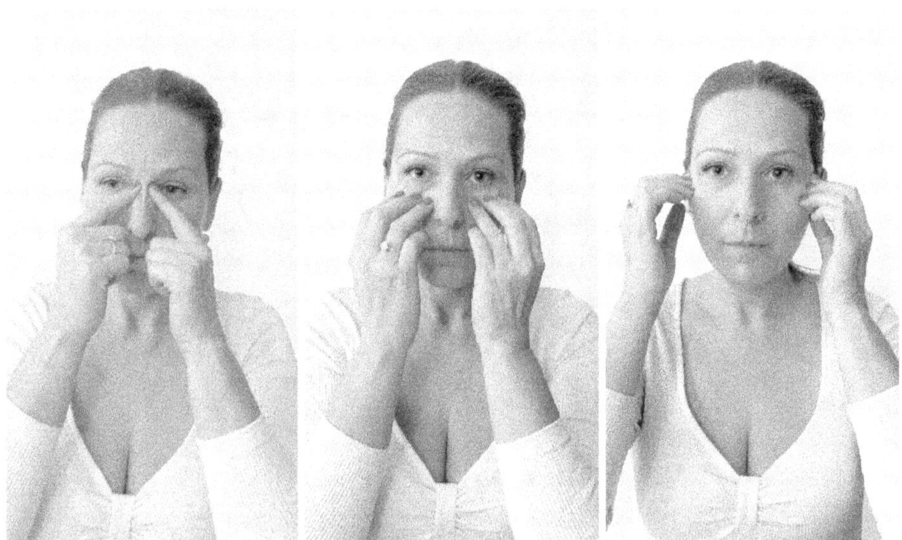

Place any finger on your tear glands, press for a few seconds and release. Continue doing this for 20-30 seconds. On the last repetition, gently massage the tear glands in a circular motion in one direction for 5-10 seconds. Lastly, start tapping under the eyes with your fingers from the inner to the outer direction for another 5-10 seconds. Repeat 5-10 times.

**Benefits:** Reduces puffiness and smoothens the area under the eyes. It nourishes the eyes and soothes dry or itchy eyes.

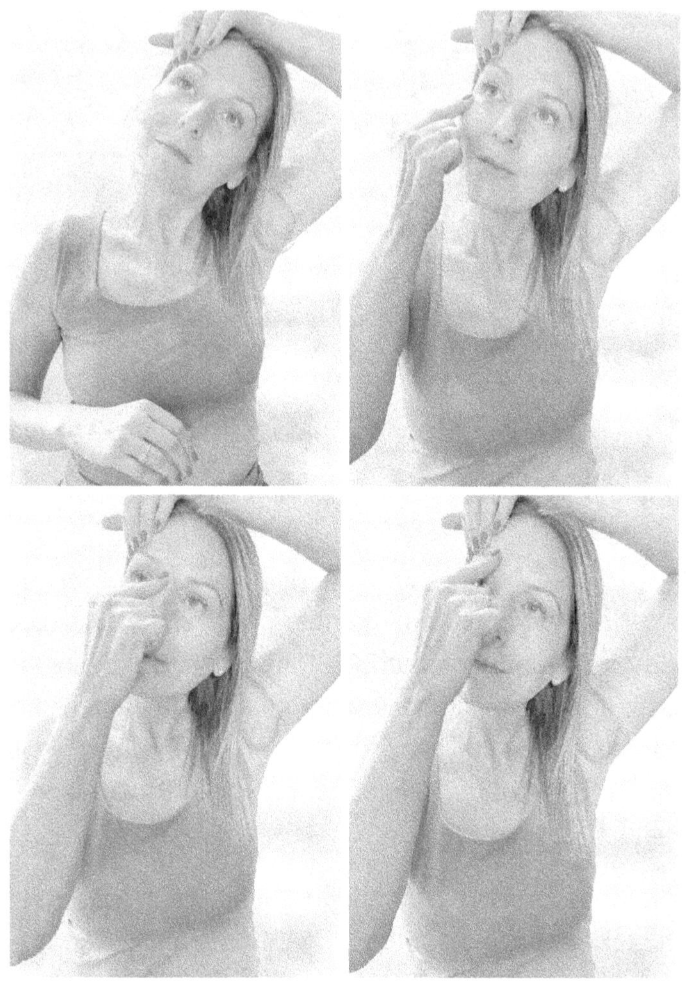

Take your right hand over your head and place your fingers above the end of your left eyebrow. Gently lift your eyebrow and with the left ring finger massage all around your eye in circular motions. Repeat 10 times. Repeat the same actions with the other eye.

Keep smiling during the practice and try to relax your mind. After finishing, tap or palm your eyes 5-10 times with your eyes closed either and release.

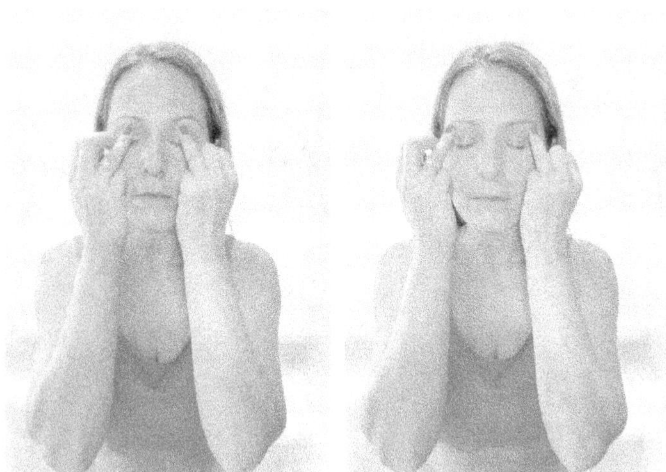

To massage your eyeballs, you do not need any moisturizer. When you massage your face, your hands are already soft and greasy from the product you used. That is sufficient for this area. Try to avoid the application of any other product, particularly a non-herbal one, since it may go into your eye and cause a burning sensation or irritation.

Close your eyes and use any finger to gently massage your eyeballs with circular motions. Do not apply any pressure while massaging them. Massage from the centre of the eyeball to all around it. Repeat 5-10 times in any direction.

Keep smiling during the practice and try to relax your mind. After finishing, either tap or palm your eyes 5-10 times with your eyes closed and release.

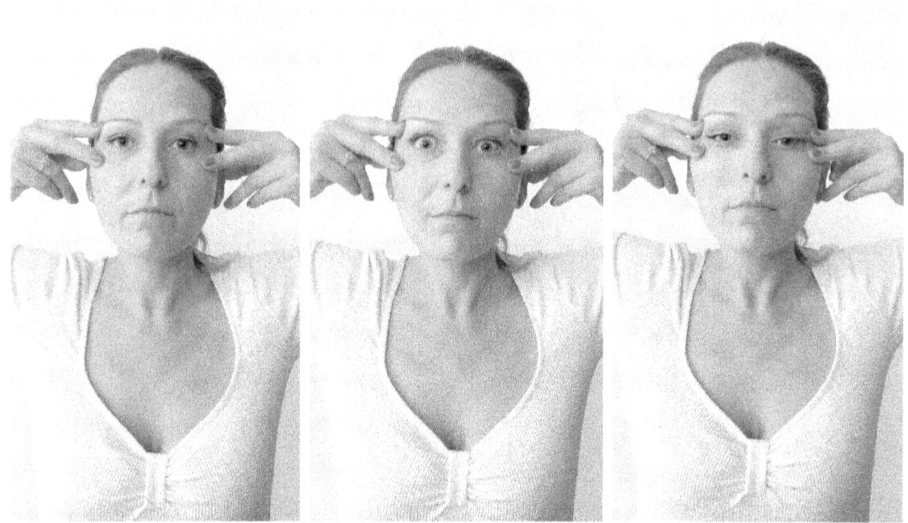

Make a V-shape with your index and middle fingers and place them at the outer corners of your eyes. Stretch your skin on an upward angle until your eyes are narrowed. Fix your gaze on a distant object and narrow your eyes further for 5 seconds. Close your eyes to release and practice 3 times.

You can do a two-finger knuckle if you like to apply more pressure. Knuckling is recommended if you want to work harder on your face to soften and reduce wrinkles around the corners of your eyes that usually appear with age.

**Benefits:** Prevents and reduces crow's feet, reduces puffiness of the eyes, tones the bags under the eyes and stimulates eye muscles.

**Precautions:** Overstretching can create extra lines. Hence, be gentle with the pressure you apply on your skin.

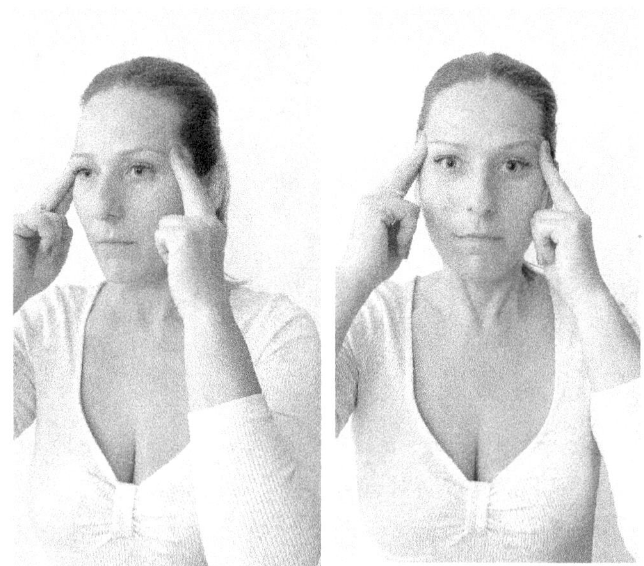

Place your index and middle fingers together on your temples. Stretch your skin upwards to lift the outer corners of your eyes. Feel the stretch on the crow's feet. Fix your gaze on a distant object and lock your eyes on it for 5 seconds. Close your eyes to release and relax for 5 seconds. Repeat 5-10 times. On the last stroke, hold the position for 3-5 seconds.

**Benefits:** Prevents and reduces crow's feet and stimulates the eye muscles.

**Precautions:** Overstretching can create extra lines; so be gentle with the pressure you apply on your skin. Remember to keep your arms up and open.

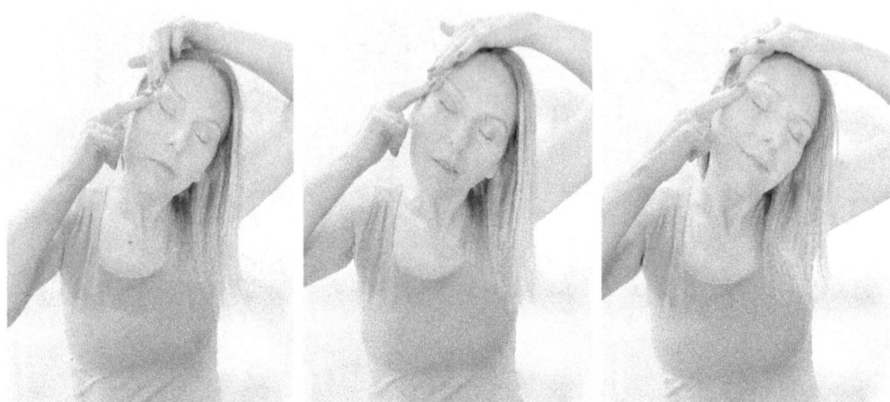

Bend your head slightly to the right. Bring your right hand over your head to hold the skin beside the end of your eyebrow. Bring the fingers of your left hand to the corner of your eye. The fingers of both hands should be beside the eye bone. With your left hand, stroke up toward your temples and hairline. Bring your right hand and hold onto the skin lifted by your left. Bring your left hand down to the original position without touching the skin. Repeat at least 5-10 times each side. On the last stroke, hold the position for 3-5 seconds.

**Benefits:** Prevents and reduces crow's feet, reduces puffiness and tones the bags under the eyes while stimulating the eye muscles.

**Precautions:** Overstretching can create extra lines; be gentle with the pressure you apply on your skin. Remember to keep your arms up and open.

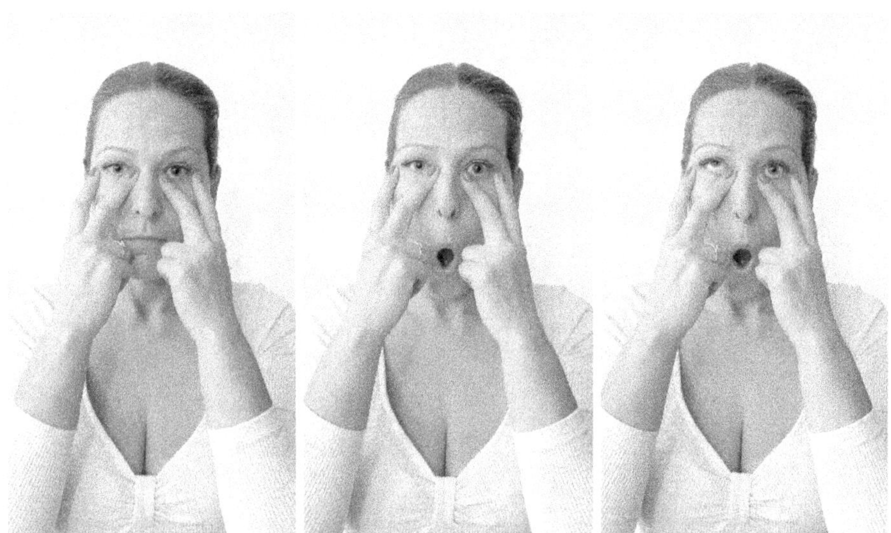

Relax your whole face. Press gently the innermost and outermost corners of your eyes with your middle/ring fingers and index fingers, respectively. Make an 'O' shape with your mouth by pressing against your teeth and your upper lip. For optimal results, fix your gaze at a 45° angle towards the sky and hold the position for 10-15 seconds and release. Close your eyes and relax for a few seconds. Repeat 5-10 times.

**Benefits:** Reduces and tones the puffiness and bags under the eyes and lengthens a rounded face.

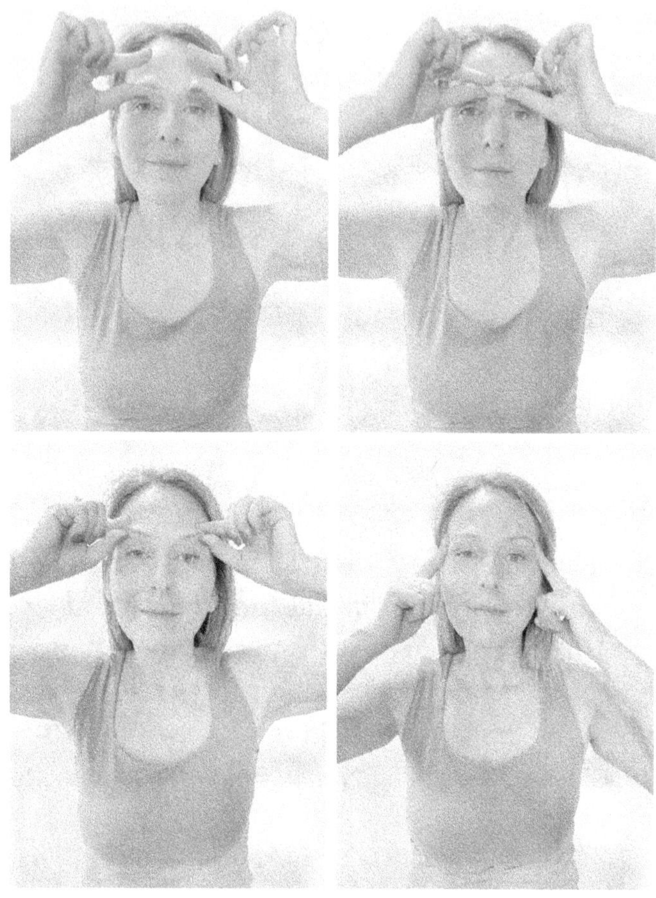

Take your index finger and thumb to pinch your eyebrows across their line. Pinch from the inner side, to the middle and towards the outside. Repeat 5-10 times. Then, stretch the eyebrows with your fingers toward the outside and up to your temples. Hold the stretch for 3-5 seconds.

**Benefits:** Helps relieve headaches. Reduces puffiness above the eyes and eyebrows. It also destresses your mind and face.

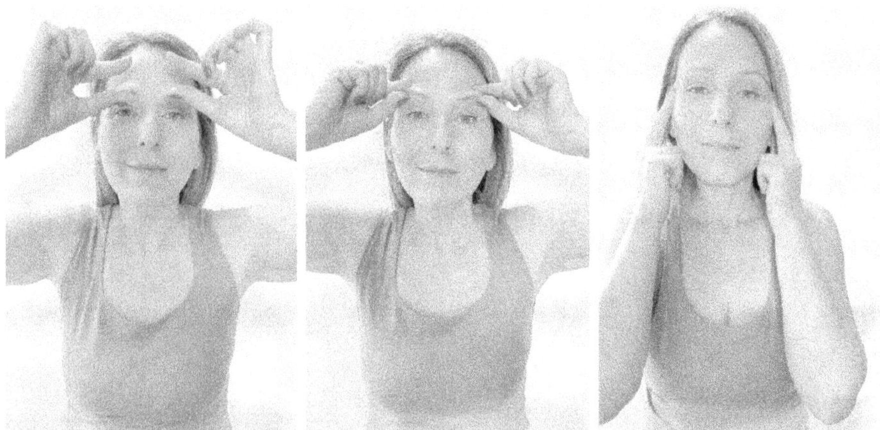

Just like pinching the eyebrows, begin from the inner side and gently pinch the eyebrows and stretch them with your fingers following their direction. Make a tiny U-turn up toward your temples from where the eyebrows end and hold for a second. Repeat 5-10 times. On the last repetition, hold the stretch on your temples with your index fingers for 5-10 seconds.

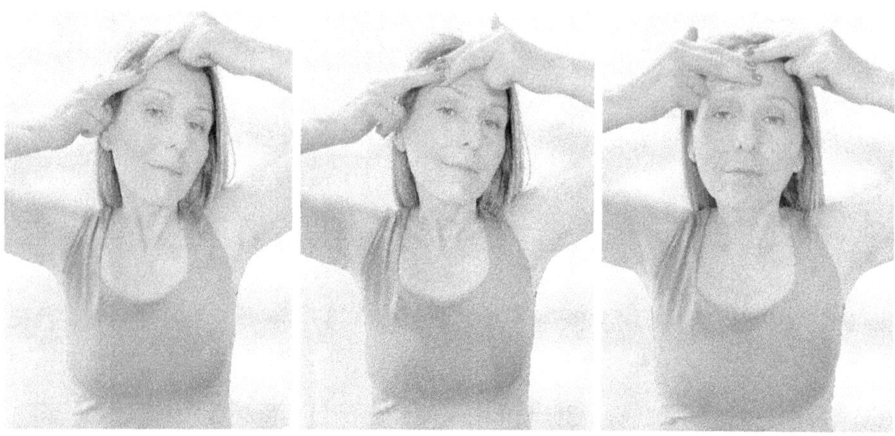

Use the index and middle fingers on each hand and start stretching your skin up and all across the forehead from the corner of your left eyebrow towards the outer side of your right eyebrow. Lift the skin with gentle pressure. With continuous motions repeat 5-10 times from side to side.

On the last stroke, hold the lifted skin for 5-10 seconds at the side you finished. Repeat 1 last time toward the opposite side and hold the skin for 5-10 seconds on that side. Take a break to relax your neck and shoulders. Breathe!

The forehead and eyes usually tend to be more tense than the other parts of our face since the stress you experience in your life leads to frowns. Massaging these areas can relax your mind and skin, tone the facial muscles, and relieve tension. It can reduce your wrinkles and stimulate the third eye which will help your focus and concentration.

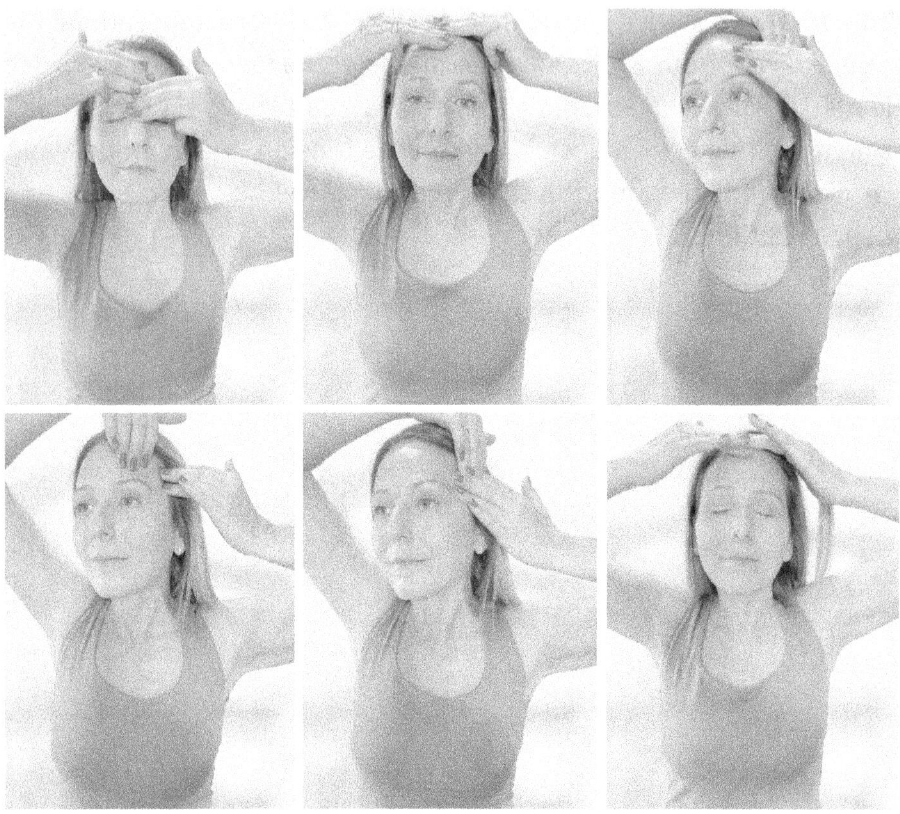

Start with the frown lines, otherwise called '11 lines' because they appear as two vertical lines between the eyebrows. Smile and place your index and middle fingers one on top of the other to lift your skin from the eyebrows to the top of the forehead. Do not drag your skin down, the motion should only be from down to up. Repeat at least 5-10 times.

On the last stroke, hold your stretched skin on the top of your forehead and by the hairline for 5-10 seconds. Do the same for the sides of your forehead.

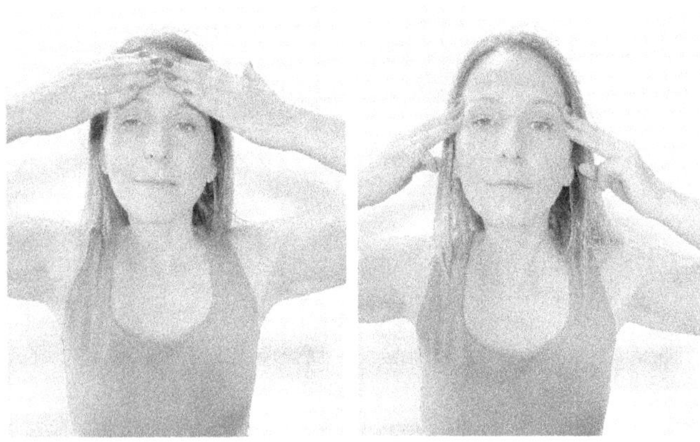

For the horizontal lines, start from the centre of your forehead with the involvement of the middle fingers of your hand. Stretch your skin gently following your eyebrow line. On every repetition, make a small U-turn up toward your temples from where they end. Repeat 5-10 times.

**Alternative:**

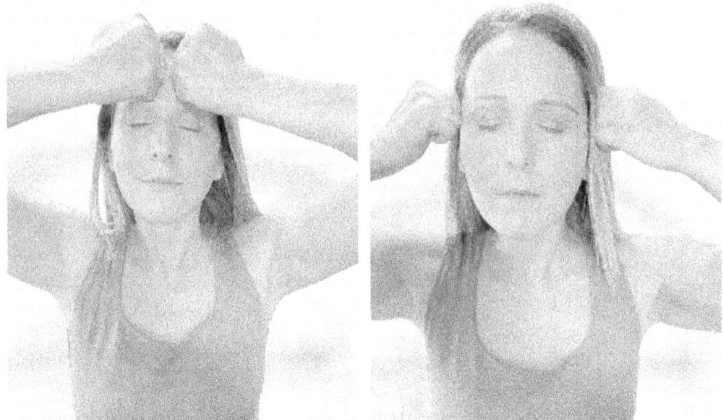

Make fists and place your hands at the centre of your forehead. Apply and maintain pressure as you slowly stroke to the sides of the forehead. Return to the centre and repeat 5-10 times. On the last repetition, apply extra pressure on your temples for 5-10 seconds and release.

# Exercise 121:   Lifting the sides

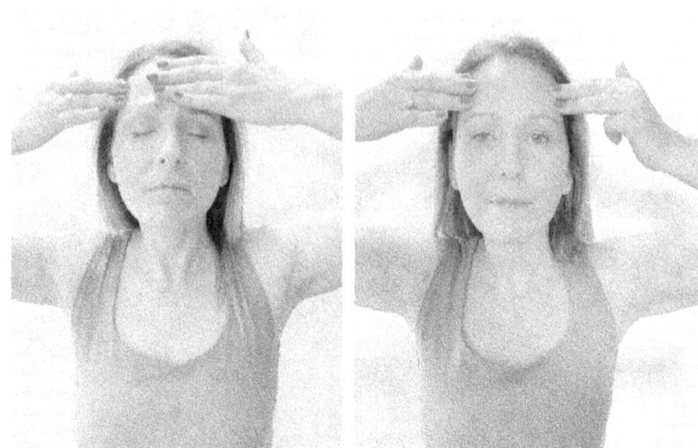

Place the middle fingers of both hands on your forehead and stroke to the sides toward your temples. Stroke to the sides in a horizontal, continuous and gentle motion. You can also hold the skin at one of the temples and stroke toward the opposite side. In this case, you will need to do the same with the other side for an equal amount of strokes. Repeat at least 5-10 times.

After completing the strokes, lift the whole face and hold for 10 seconds with normal breathing. Release and relax with 2-3 deep breaths.

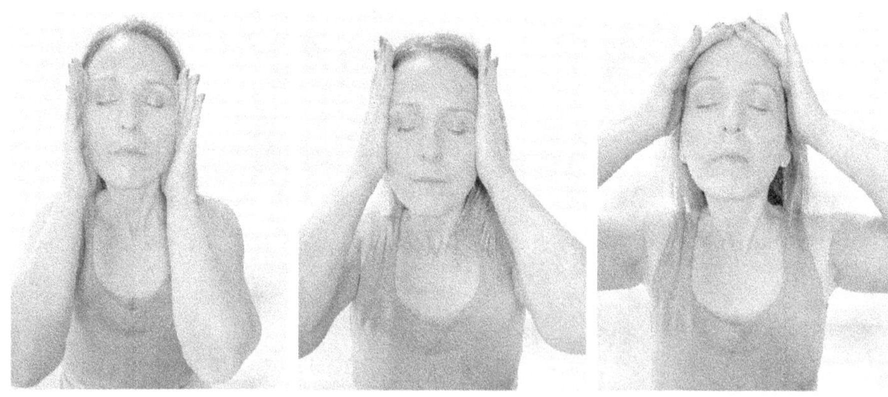

## Exercise 122:    Acupressure points on the forehead

**Option A:**

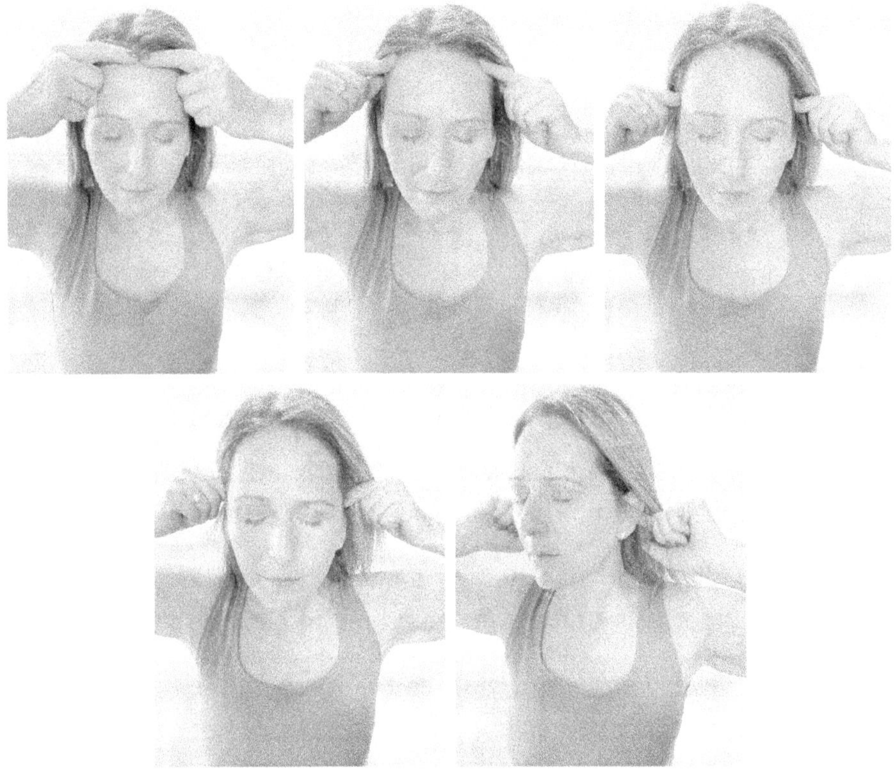

Use your index fingers and start from the centre of your hairline, press
and release continuously across the hairline. Slide your fingers to the
back of the ear to complete the stroke at the bottom of the ear. Repeat
5-10 times.

**Option B:**

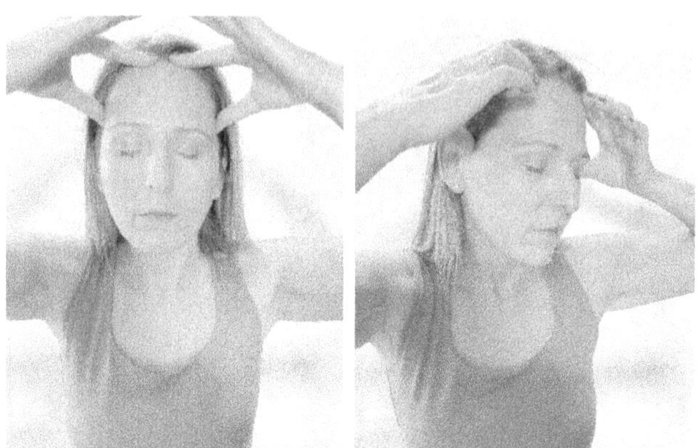

Place your thumbs beside the top of your ear and your index fingers at the centre of your hairline. Slightly stretch, press and release continuously across your hairline, starting from the centre and up to the ears. Repeat 5-10 times.

**Note:** If you like, you can do the same over your entire scalp to stimulate the pores of the hair for healthier and longer hair.

**Benefits:** Relieves headaches, relaxes the forehead, removes tension and prevents and lifts wrinkles.

To finish your facial massage, continue with the following techniques not only to finish lifting your skin but also to relax your skin, muscles and mind. Alternatively, this is a quick facial massage for everyday use.

Practise each step only once with your eyes closed. Before you begin, take a few slow and deep breaths. Relax your body, particularly your shoulders, relax your face, and relax your mind. With gentle pressure:

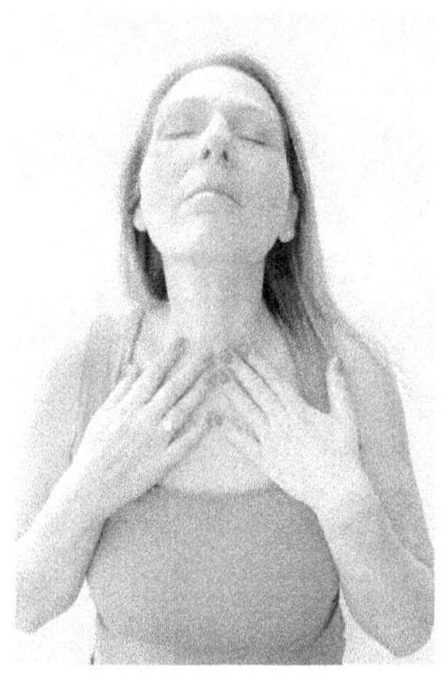

Place your hands on your chest area and gently lift your skin sideways toward your armpits. Hold the stretch for 3-5 seconds.

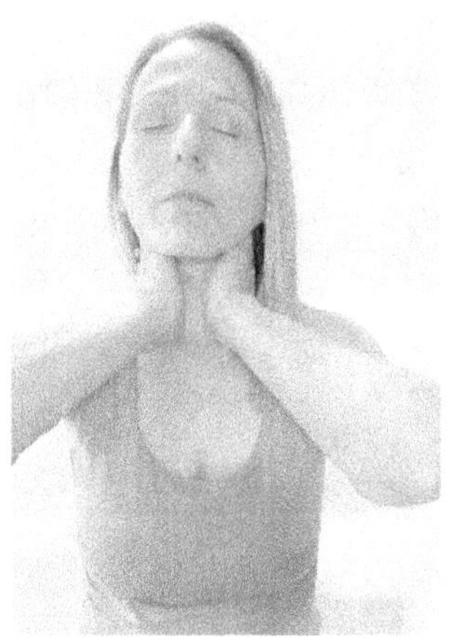

Place your hands on your neck to stroke the back of the neck. Hold the stretch for 3-5 seconds.

Tones the skin of your throat.

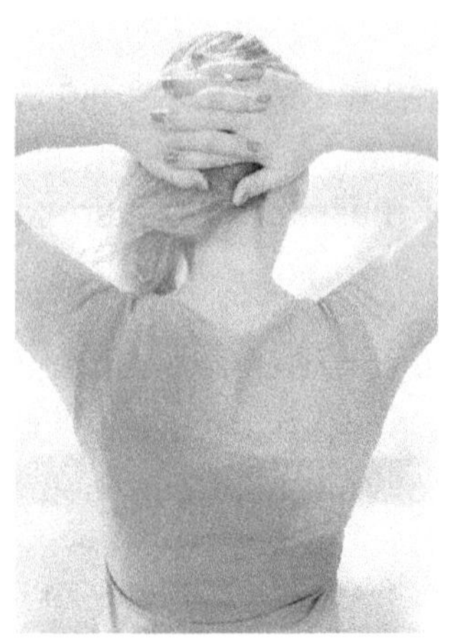

Slide your hands up and interlock them at the centre behind your head.

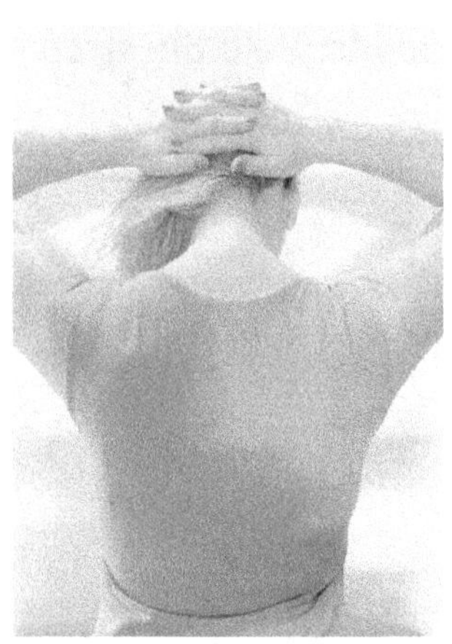

With your fingers interlocked, gently push your head to look down and stretch the back of the neck. Hold the stretch for 3-5 seconds.

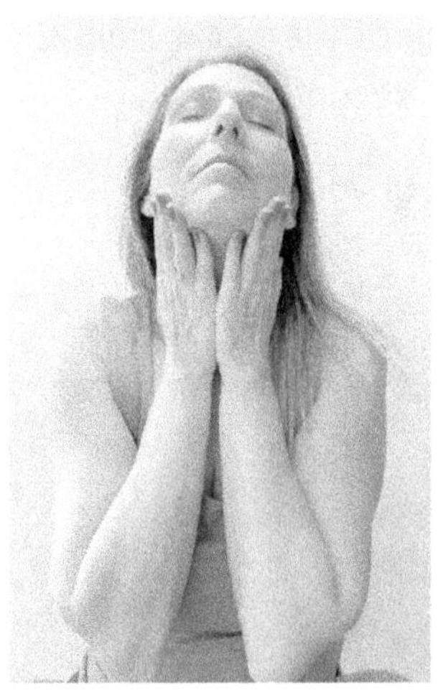

Bring your head back up to the neutral position. Take your hands back in front of your neck and stroke them up to your chin and jaw. Hold the stretch for 3-5 seconds.

Lifts the double chin.

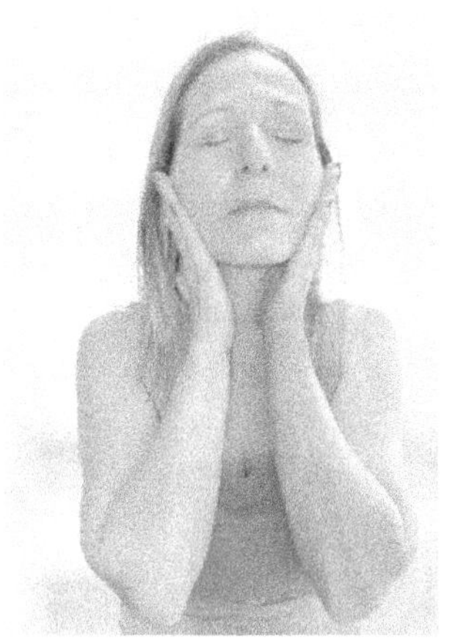

Continue to stroke from the sides and under your jawline up toward your ears. Hold the stretch for 3-5 seconds.

Lifts the sides of the double chin and shapes the jawline.

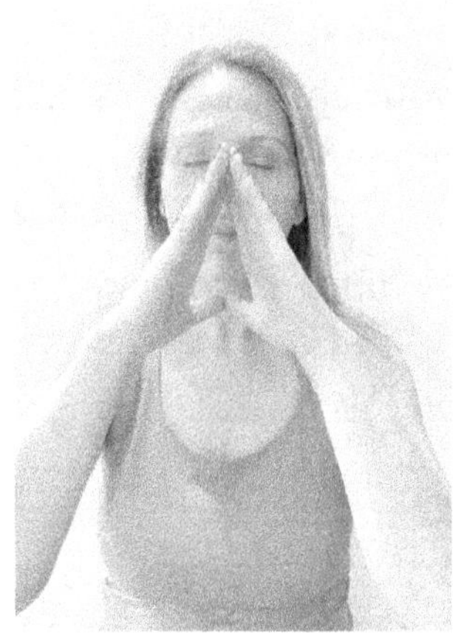

Bring your palms to make a triangle with your fingers by your nose area. This is your starting pose for strokes that go from the front of the face to the sides.

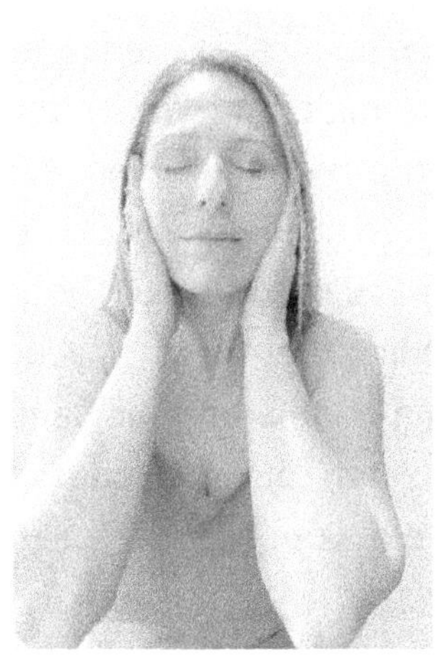

From the starting pose, stretch the lower side of your cheeks by making a U-shaped motion. Hold for 3-5 seconds with your index fingers beside your ears with your pinky fingers holding the stretch.

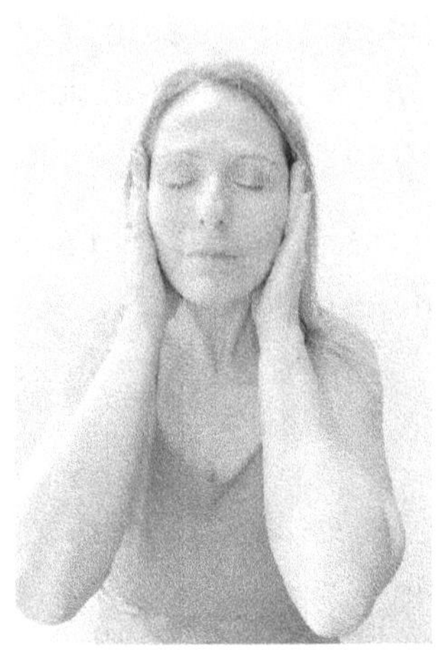

From starting pose, stretch the middle of your cheeks by making a U-shaped motion. Hold for 3-5 seconds with your index fingers on your ears and your ring fingers holding the stretch.

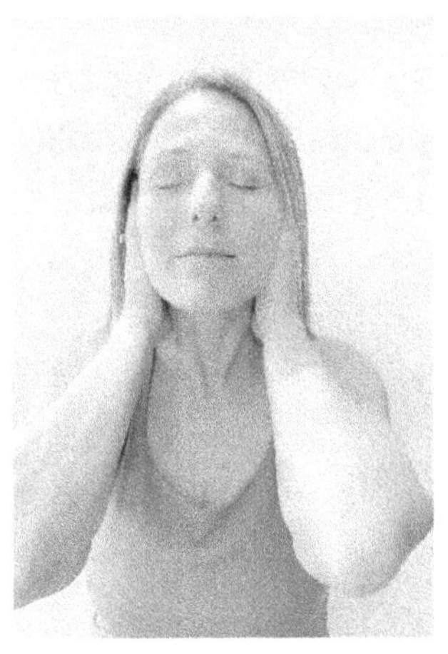

From starting pose, stretch the upper side of your cheeks by making a U-shaped motion. Hold for 3-5 seconds with your palm on your ears and your pinky fingers holding the stretch.

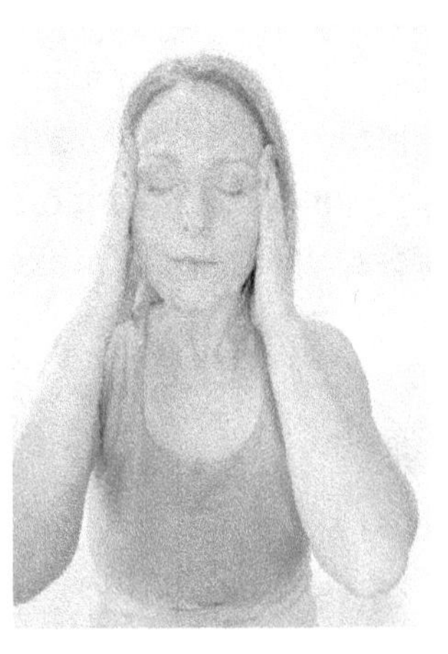

From starting pose, stretch the upper cheeks with the middle of your palm and the skin on top of your eyes and eyebrows with your fingertips. Hold the position for 3-5 seconds with your ring fingers holding the stretch at your temples and the middle of your palm holding the stretch of your cheeks and the corners of your mouth.

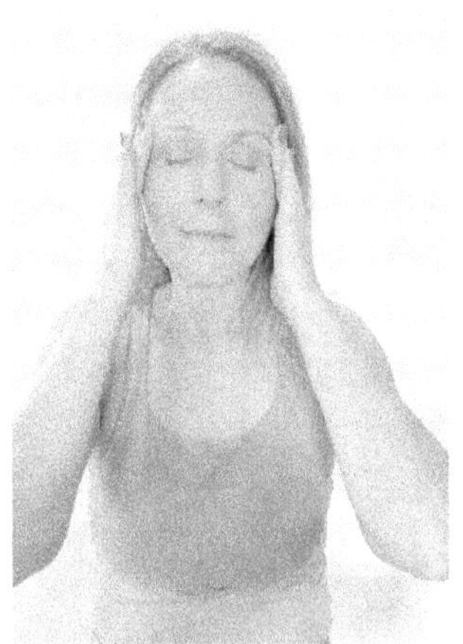

Do the same as the previous step with your fingers only around your eyes. Stroke and hold the stretch for 3-5 seconds with your index and middle fingers at your temples.

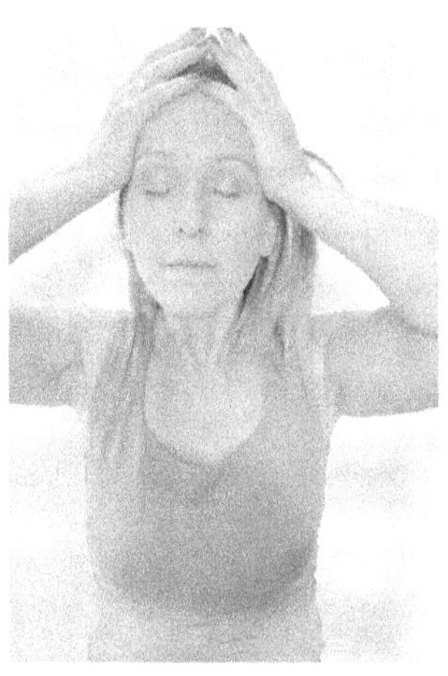

Place your thumbs on top of your ears and make a pyramid with your fingers starting under your eyebrows. Maintain the position of the hands and stroke up towards your hairline. Hold the stretch on your hairline with your pinky fingers for 3-5 seconds.

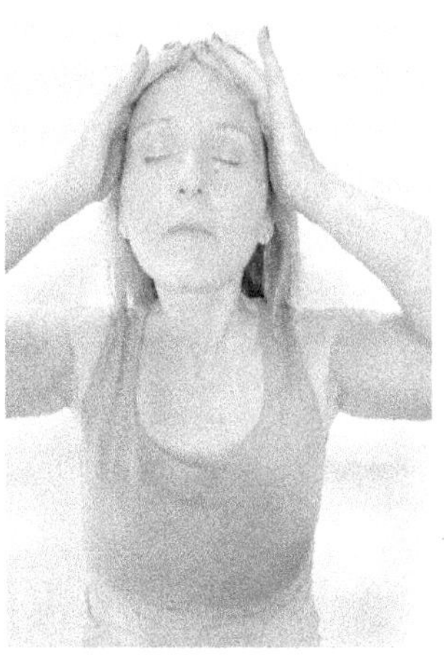

Stroke your fingers towards your crown by applying some pressure for 3-5 seconds. Feel the relaxation. Move the fingers behind the head to the centre and do the same.

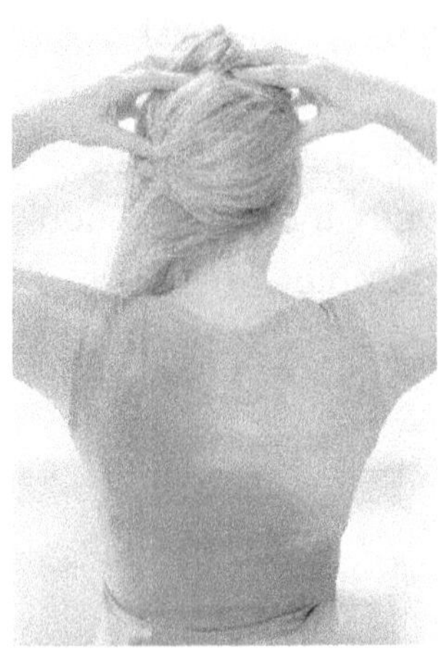

Open your fingers and in random motions apply gentle pressure in various parts of your head for at least 30 seconds.

Stimulates the pores of your hair to help them glow and grow longer and reduces stress and anxiety.

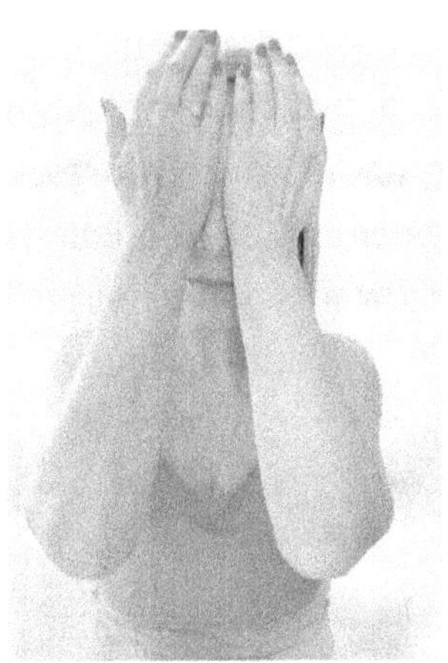

To finish this massage, cup your eyes with your palms and by following the palming exercise. Keep breathing. Slowly open your eyes.

Massaging the ears relaxes the nerves that vibrate through the whole body. It also stimulates the senses and the skin to improve its quality, reduces muscle pain and helps relieve headaches and migraines, boosts blood circulation and gives a sense of relaxation and happiness!

The points in front of the ear and back of the ear are useful points for facial relaxation.

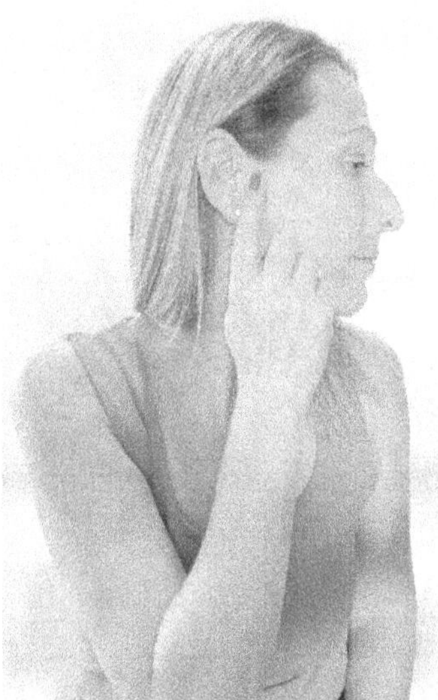 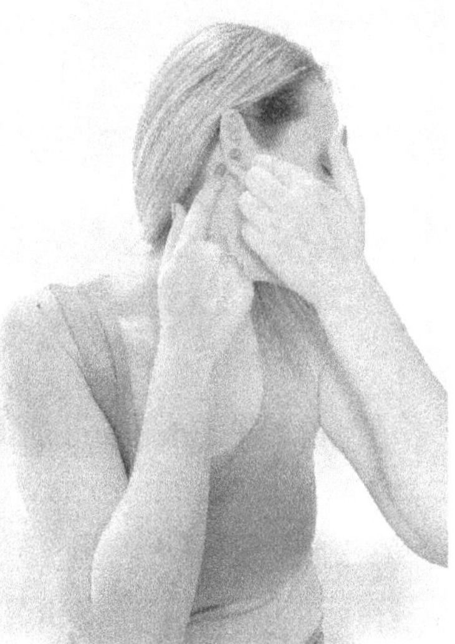

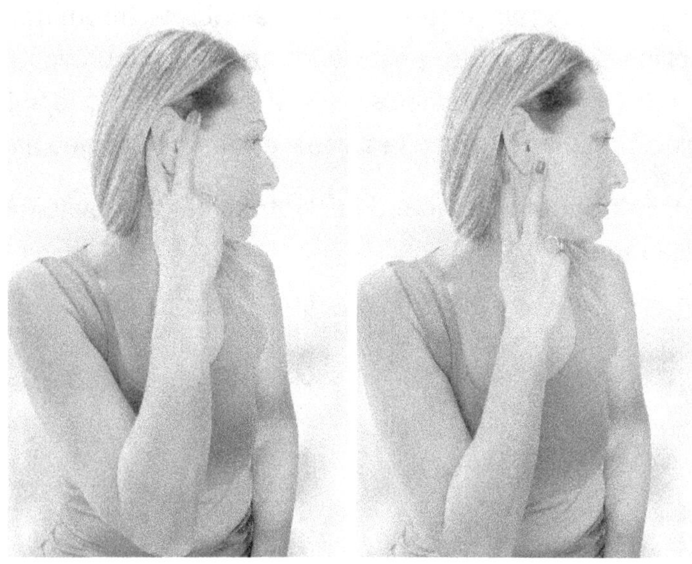

Make a V-shape with your fingers. Place your middle fingers on the inner side of the face and the index fingers on the back of the ear. Stroke with normal speed and slide up to your ears as well as down to your jawbone. Practise both sides at the same time to maintain facial symmetry. Repeat 20-30 times.

**Benefits:** It is a relaxing technique and stimulates the ear muscles and nerves. It also relieves ear congestion, ringing in the ears and pain in the jaw.

**Note:** To help reduce the sides of the double chin, practice only upward strokes with your index finger starting the movement from the jaw bone.

## Exercise 125:   Pinching the ears

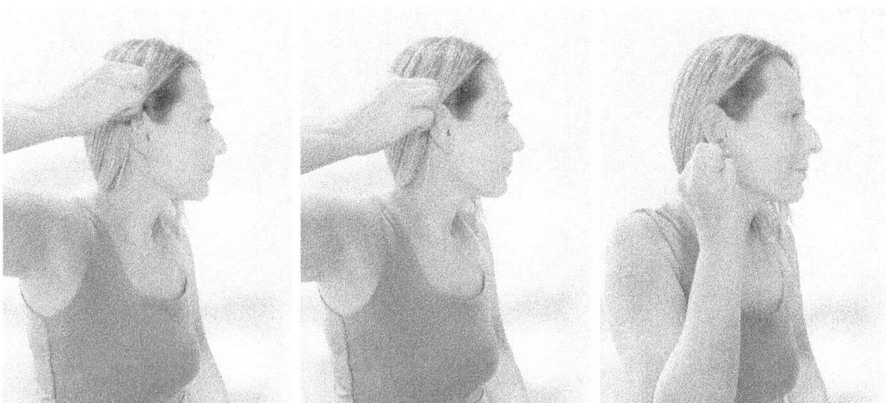

Pinch one ear at a time with your fingers starting from the top down to the outer lid of the ear and the lobe. When you reach your ear lobe, press for 3-5 seconds and release. Repeat 5-10 times from top to down.

**Note:** The ear lobe is considered to be the brain of the body since in acupressure language it is connected to the brain. This practice will stimulate the brain.

## Exercise 126:  Stimulating nerves in the ears

**Step 1:**

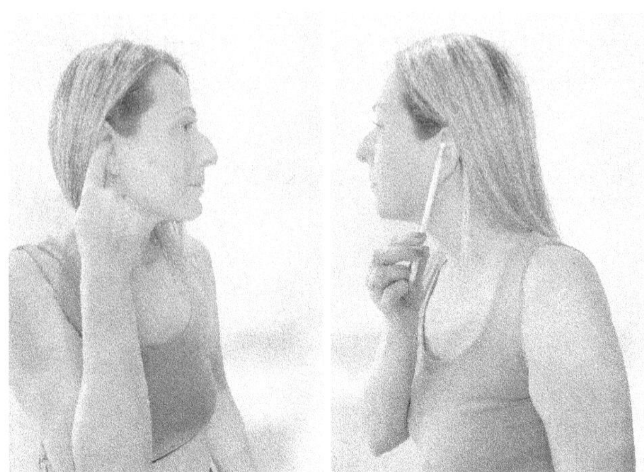

Press the upper concha (located at the top of the small cartilage) with your index finger for 10 seconds and release. Repeat 3-5 times.

**Step 2:**

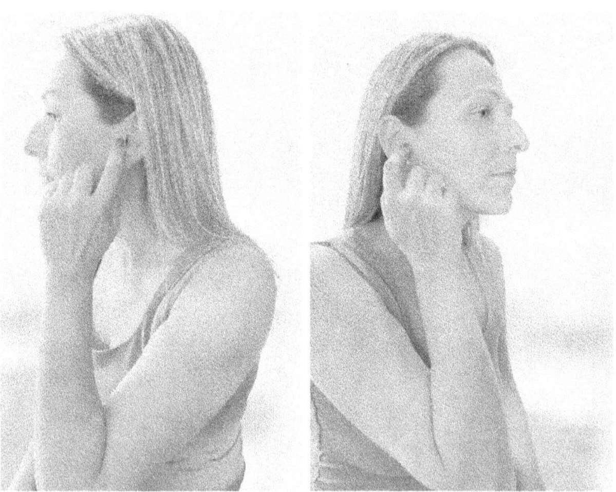

Either pinch or press your tragus (the small lobe at the centre of the outer ear) for 3-5 seconds at a time and release. Repeat 5-10 times on each ear.

# Relaxation after Massage

After completing your massage, you can add some meditation time to relax your mind and skin. If this is new to you, record the following text and play it back every time you need to relax and stimulate your senses.

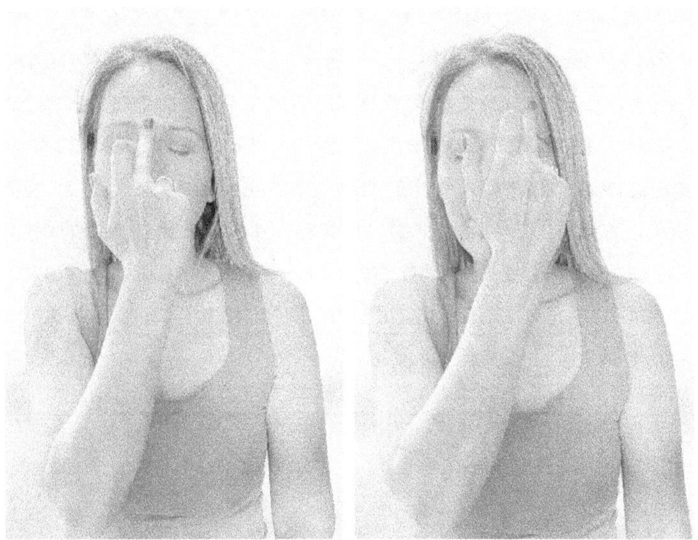

Choose a comfortable seated position, sit in a chair, or lie down. Take your finger and place it between your eyebrows at the Ajna (third-eye) Chakra. Smile during this practice. Start with 10 small circular motions between the eyebrows. Then make 10 bigger circles to cover the corners of the eyebrows. Think of a whirlpool as you progress with your movements. Keep calm and relax during this massage with your eyes closed. Keep breathing normally. Then make 10 bigger circles to cover the centre of your forehead. Be yourself and remember all the good memories that make you smile. Smile with them now and every day. Remove all excess thinking and any negative thoughts you may have. Connect your motion with your breath. Smile and inhale on the upward motion while exhaling on the downward motion. After that, make 10 bigger circles to cover your forehead area. Visualize what you need, what you desire, what you want, and what you wish. Breathe in nice thoughts and breathe out anything that is bothering you. Breathe in health into your mind and body and breathe out any pain and tension you may have. Breathe in and feel positive and breathe out and remove any possible obstacles.

After you finish, keep your eyes closed and try to see what colour comes to you with your third eye. Focus on that colour for as long as you can, so that you can eliminate all thoughts from your mind for these few moments. Shut down your thinking process and relax your mind. As you see this colour fading away, palm your hands to generate enough heat and cup your eyes for a few seconds to transfer that heat back to your body. Transfer that heat all over your face, front and back neck, shoulders, chest and rib cage, wherever your hands can travel. When you are ready, open your eyes. Keep smiling! Keep breathing! Keep being positive!

Drink some water. Finish your massage by tapping all over your face, head, neck and chest areas.

# Meditation Colours

A quick guide of the colours you may visualize and their meaning:

## Meditation Colors

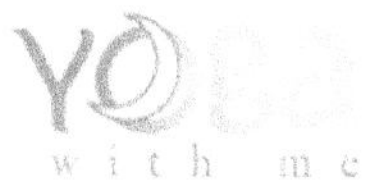

| | | |
|---|---|---|
| **Black** | : | Power, Control, Secrets, Loneliness |
| **Blue** | : | Trust, Loyalty, Communication, Stubbornness |
| **Green** | : | Inner Peace, Forgiveness, Compassion |
| **Orange** | : | Happiness, Energy, Adventure, Independence |
| **Pink** | : | Unconditional Love, Romanticism, Thoughtfulness |
| **Purple** | : | Imagination, Spirituality, Consciousness |
| **Red** | : | Energy, Strength, Passion, Anger |
| **White** | : | Intuitions, Purity |
| **Yellow** | : | Logic, Creativity, Confidence, Ego |

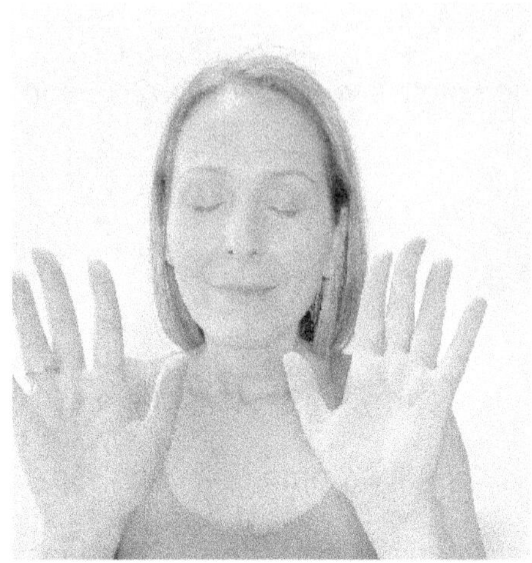

When you think that you have had enough, follow the 'Face Yoga With Me' community to learn all about upcoming events and news.

www.yogawithme.co.in

Contact me directly at:

https://www.instagram.com/yogawithmeglobal/
OR
https://www.facebook.com/yogawithmeglobal/

www.ingramcontent.com/pod-product-compliance
Lightning Source LLC
Chambersburg PA
CBHW060911140726
47996CB00001B/199